Pocket Anatomy of
Cerebrovascular Imaging
and Topography

Pocket Anatomy of Cerebrovascular Imaging and Topography

Dong-Eog Kim

Dongguk University Hospital, Korea
& Massachusetts General Hospital, USA

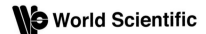 **World Scientific**

NEW JERSEY · LONDON · SINGAPORE · BEIJING · SHANGHAI · HONG KONG · TAIPEI · CHENNAI · TOKYO

Published by

World Scientific Publishing Co. Pte. Ltd.

5 Toh Tuck Link, Singapore 596224

USA office: 27 Warren Street, Suite 401-402, Hackensack, NJ 07601

UK office: 57 Shelton Street, Covent Garden, London WC2H 9HE

Library of Congress Cataloging-in-Publication Data

Names: Kim, Dong-Eog, author.

Title: Pocket anatomy of cerebrovascular imaging and topography / Dong-Eog Kim.

Description: New Jersey : World Scientific, [2020] | Includes index.

Identifiers: LCCN 2020008814 | ISBN 9789811209369 (hardcover) |
    ISBN 9789811211447 (paperback) |
    ISBN 9789811209376 (ebook for institutions) |
    ISBN 9789811209383 (ebook for individuals)

Subjects: MESH: Brain--anatomy & histology | Cerebral Arteries--anatomy &
    histology | Brain--diagnostic imaging | Cerebral Arteries--diagnostic
    imaging | Atlas | Handbook

Classification: LCC QP376 | NLM WL 39 | DDC 612.8/2--dc23

LC record available at https://lccn.loc.gov/2020008814

British Library Cataloguing-in-Publication Data

A catalogue record for this book is available from the British Library.

For any available supplementary material, please visit
https://www.worldscientific.com/worldscibooks/10.1142/11528#t=suppl

Printed in Singapore

Contents

Foreword

Neurologists, neuroscientists, and neurosurgeons have always been accused of having an obsessional focus on anatomy - neuroanatomy. The brain is unique and different from other organs. In the liver, kidney, lung, and in virtually every other systemic organ, one part looks like and functions like any other. In the brain various functions are well localized to specific brain regions and the gross and microscopic anatomy differ in each region. When I was a Neurology resident and later a stroke fellow in the 1960s, the only available way to localize a brain lesion was from the clinical symptoms and neurological signs. I wanted to understand how each part of the brain functioned so that I could help patients understand and recover from their clinical abnormalities. If I could localize the area of the brain involved, and I knew the arteries and veins that supplied and drained that region, I could estimate the likelihood of various pathologies affecting those vessels. Vascular images could only be obtained by injecting large volumes of dye after the neck arteries were individually punctured, a procedure with considerable hazards. Neurosurgeons during that period needed to know exactly where a tumor, abscess or other surgical lesion was located in order to remove the appropriate skull region and so gain approach to the lesion. Of course, they did not want to remove brain tissue that would disable the patient. They also relied on clinical symptoms and signs.

When CT became available during the 1970s, and subsequent generation CT scanners became more diagnostic, a quantum leap occurred in clinical localization of brain lesions. The advent of MRI scanning during the 1980s led to even better definition of brain anatomy and brain dysfunction. Subsequent technological innovations led to relatively non-invasive vascular imaging - CT and MR angiography, and digital subtraction techniques led to less hazardous and better pictures after directly injecting arteries and veins. Neurologists and neurosurgeons now have excellent technology available to localize brain lesions and their vascular supply. They could also define much better the location, nature, and severity of vascular abnormalities.

After the turn of the century, a major change occurred in neurosurgery and in vascular neurology. More and more treatment of vascular lesions - blocked arteries, aneurysms, arterio-venous malformations, and brain hemorrhages were treated through the vascular system by interventionalists. These physicians were, at first, mostly neurosurgeons, but later neuroradiologists and neurologists began to perform interventional treatment. The effectiveness of many of these treatments depended highly on their being performed quickly and efficiently. Doctors need a readily available user-friendly resource that they could go to that would yield accurate brain and vascular anatomy information quickly and easily.

Dr. Dong-Eon Kim has created that needed resource in this Atlas. The pictures within the atlas are very clear and easily studied and interpreted. The Atlas begins with detailed axial sections of the brain that show in black and white and in color various cortical and deep structures at various clearly designated levels of section. The next chapter shows the anterior and posterior circulation arteries, and their usual supply and watershed regions, first on axial MRI sections and then on CT scans. This is followed by a chapter on arterial topography supply and watershed zones on coronal MRI sections at various levels. Later chapters show images created during MR angiography and venography and during digital subtraction angiography and vessel wall MRI imaging. The last sections contain examples of visual estimation of the burden of white matter ischemic pathology and of infarct volumes on MRI sections.

This atlas has been meticulously researched and elegantly produced. The figures are of very high quality and easy to interpret. It provides ready access to clinicians-neurologists, neuroradiologists and neurosurgeons, and to neuroscience researchers about brain and vascular anatomy irrespective of which technological modality is chosen.

Louis R. Caplan MD

Professor Neurology, Harvard University

Preface

This atlas provides anatomical knowledge of cerebral vascular imaging and topography, which is not only important for neurological or neurosurgical practice, but also useful for neurovascular or neuroscience research.

I began to think about vascular territorial mapping using a large set of clinical MRI datasets, the key content of this book, when I was working as a post-doc radiology research fellow at the Center for Molecular Imaging Research at Massachusetts General Hospital from 2002 to 2005. Prior to joining the institute, I had finished my neurology residency and stroke fellowship at Seoul National University Hospital. During my training years, I experienced the importance of vascular anatomy on a daily basis. How nice it would have been had this book been in my pocket during those years!

These days, many people prefer electronic books to paper books. However, printed books are better for skimming and looking up images, as well as highlighting, drawing, and making notes here and there. This "paper" book has blank pages for your own (hand-writing) contribution to modify it to a uniquely customized version, i.e., the one and only book in the world. Please, do not forget that this "portable" book, which easily fits in your pocket, and does not need electric power.

I thank all the co-authors for their valuable contributions and dedication. Without their time and effort, completing this book would not have been possible. All images are from patients or volunteers, whom I deeply thank. I also thank the publishers of World Scientific, particularly Ms. Sook Cheng Lim, for supporting the idea and concept of book from the beginning and providing advice at all stages during the process of preparing the book. I thank my friend (and teacher) Eng Lo, Director of Neuroprotection Research Laboratory and Professor of Radiology at Harvard Medical School, for supporting the book proposal and introducing me to the publisher. I thank Dr. Jung E Park, Su-Kyoung Lee, and Da-Hye Heo for their help in preparing topography images. I must acknowledge Hyun Jin Sim for teaching me watercolor painting and pencil art; she took a rain check on preparing the cover design, thus letting me do it all by myself!

I also thank my talented friend, Dawid Schellingerhout, Professor, Departments of Radiology and Experimental Diagnostic Imaging at M.D. Anderson Cancer Center, for having done imaging science with me for 15 years. Together we have co-authored more than 30 articles, some of which are key references of this book.

Lastly, I would like to thank my dear parents and parents-in-law, my wife and best friend, Yun-Young, and sons, June Sup and Bo Sup, for their love and blessings.

Dong-Eog Kim

PART

1

[Memo]

Supratentorial Brain Anatomy

Su-Kyoung Lee, BSc and Dong-Eog Kim, MD, PhD

Twelve MNI ICBM 152 T1 template images were selected: z = -16, -10, -4, 2, 9, 15, 21, 27, 33, 39, 45, and 52 mm from the anterior commissure – posterior commissure line.

1. VS Fonov, AC Evans, K Botteron, CR Almli, RC McKinstry, DL Collins and BDCG. Unbiased average age-appropriate atlases for pediatric studies. *NeuroImage* 2011; 54 : 313 - 327. ISSN 1053–8119, DOI: 10.1016/j.neuroimage.2010.07.033

2. VS Fonov, AC Evans, RC McKinstry, CR Almli and DL Collins. Unbiased nonlinear average age-appropriate brain templates from birth to adulthood. *NeuroImage* 2009; 47 : S102, Organization for Human Brain Mapping 2009 Annual Meeting, DOI: http://dx.doi.org/10.1016/S1053-8119(09)70884-5

z = -16 mm from the Anterior Commissure – Posterior Commissure Line

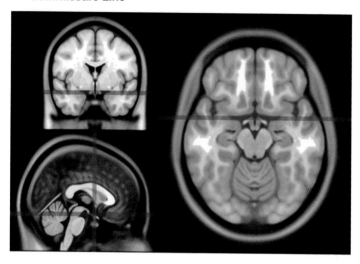

z = -10 mm from the Anterior Commissure – Posterior Commissure Line

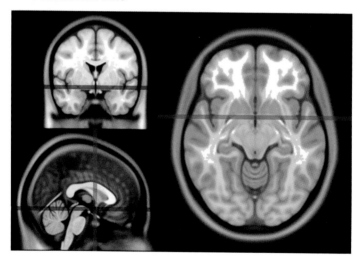

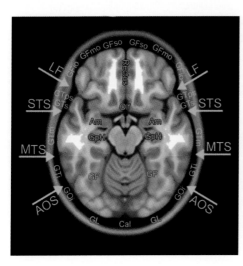

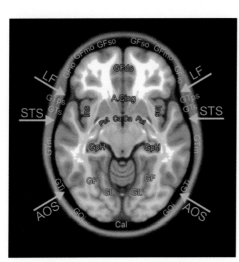

A. Cing: anterior cingulate gyrus
Am: amygdala
AOS: anterior occipital sulcus
Ca: caudate
Cal: calcarine gyrus
GF: fusiform gyrus
GFdo: middle pre-fronto-orbital gyrus
GFio: orbital part of the inferior frontal gyrus
GFmo: orbital part of the middle frontal gyrus
GFso: orbital part of the superior frontal gyrus
GL: lingual gyrus
GOi: inferior occipital gyrus
GpH: parahippocampal gyrus
GTi: inferior temporal gyrus
GTm: middle temporal gyrus
GTps: temporal pole
GTs: superior temporal gyrus
Ins: insula
LF: lateral fissure
MTS: middle temporal sulcus
Olf: olfactory gyrus
Put: putamen
Rectus: gyrus rectus
STS: superior temporal sulcus

z = - 4 mm from the Anterior Commissure – Posterior Commissure Line

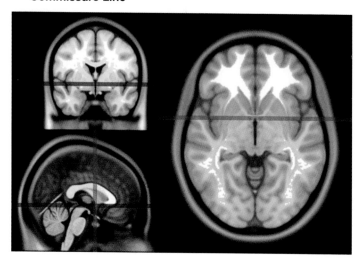

z = 2 mm from the Anterior Commissure – Posterior Commissure Line

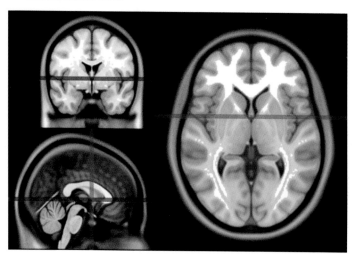

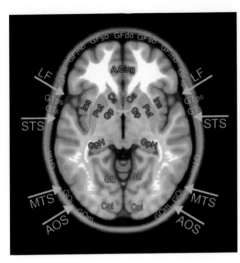

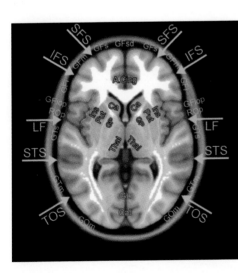

A. Cing: anterior cingulate gyrus
AOS: anterior occipital sulcus
Ca: caudate
Cal: calcarine gyrus
GFdo: middle pre-fronto-orbital gyrus
GFi: inferior frontal gyrus
GFio: orbital part of the inferior frontal gyrus
GFiop: opercular part of the inferior frontal gyrus
GFm: middle frontal gyrus
GFmo: orbital part of the middle frontal gyrus
GFs: superior frontal gyrus
GFsd: superior part of the medial frontal gyrus
GFso: orbital part of the superior frontal gyrus
GL: lingual gyrus
GOi: inferior occipital gyrus
GOm: middle occipital gyrus
Gp: globus pallidus
GpH: parahippocampal gyrus
GTm: middle temporal gyrus
GTps: temporal pole
GTs: superior temporal gyrus
IFS: inferior frontal sulcus
Ins: insula
LF: lateral fissure
MTS: middle temporal sulcus
Put: putamen
ROp: rolandic operculum
SFS: superior frontal sulcus
STS: superior temporal sulcus
Thal: thalamus
TOS: temporooccipital sulcus

z = 9 mm from the Anterior Commissure – Posterior Commissure Line

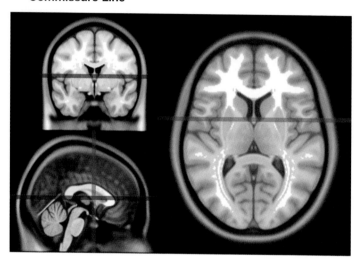

z = 15 mm from the Anterior Commissure – Posterior Commissure Line

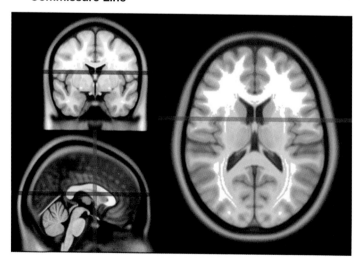

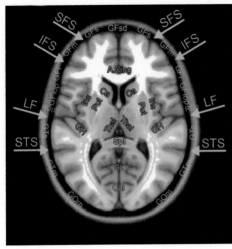

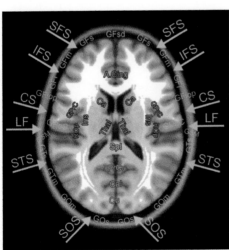

A. Cing: anterior cingulate gyrus

Ca: caudate

Cal: calcarine gyrus

CS: central sulcus

Cu: cuneus

GFi: inferior frontal gyrus

GFiop: opercular part of the inferior frontal gyrus

GFm: middle frontal gyrus

GFs: superior frontal gyrus

GFsd: superior part of the medial frontal gyrus

GH: Heschl gyrus

GL: lingual gyrus

GOm: middle occipital gyrus

GOs: superior occipital gyrus

GPoC: postcentral gyrus

GPrC: precentral gyrus

GSM: supramarginal gyrus

GTm: middle temporal gyrus

GTs: superior temporal gyrus

IFS: inferior frontal sulcus

Ins: insula

LF: lateral fissure

PrCu: precuneus

Put: putamen

ROp: rolandic operculum

SFS: superior frontal sulcus

SOS: superior occipital sulcus

Spl: splenium

STS: superior temporal sulcus

Thal: thalamus

z = 21 mm from the Anterior Commissure – Posterior Commissure Line

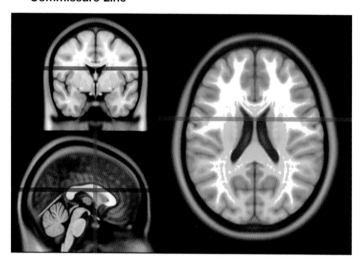

z = 27 mm from the Anterior Commissure – Posterior Commissure Line

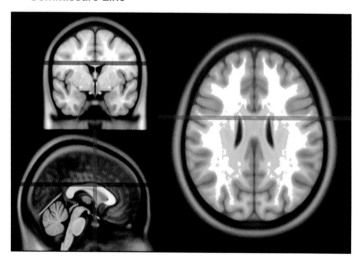

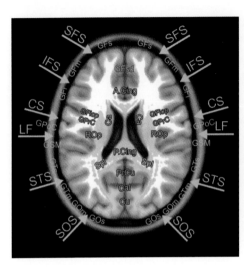

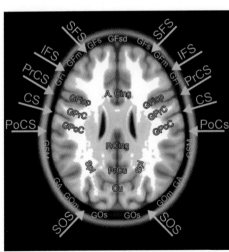

A. Cing: anterior cingulate gyrus
Ca: caudate
Cal: calcarine gyrus
CS: central sulcus
Cu: cuneus
GA: angular gyrus
GFiop: opercular part of the inferior frontal gyrus
GFi: inferior frontal gyrus
GFm: middle frontal gyrus
GFs: superior frontal gyrus
GFsd: superior part of the medial frontal gyrus
GOm: middle occipital gyrus
GOs: superior occipital gyrus
GPoC: postcentral gyrus
GPrC: precentral gyrus
GSM: supramarginal gyrus
GTm: middle temporal gyrus
GTs: superior temporal gyrus
IFS: inferior frontal sulcus
LF: lateral fissure
P. Cing: posterior cingulate gyrus
PoCS: postcentral sulcus
PrCS: precentral sulcus
PrCu: precuneus
ROp: rolandic operculum
SFS: superior frontal sulcus
SOS: superior occipital sulcus
Spl: splenium
STS: superior temporal sulcus

z = 33 mm from the Anterior Commissure – Posterior Commissure Line

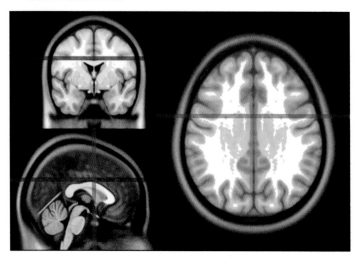

z = 39 mm from the Anterior Commissure – Posterior Commissure Line

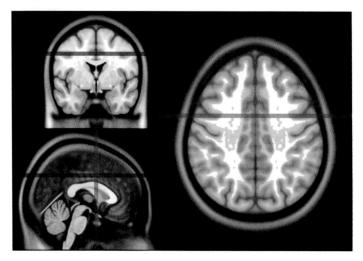

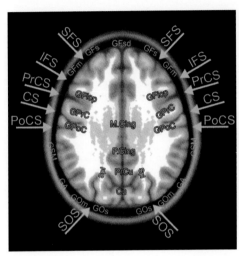

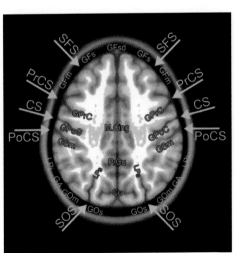

CS: central sulcus
Cu: cuneus
GA: angular gyrus
GFiop: opercular part of the inferior frontal gyrus
GFm: middle frontal gyrus
GFs: superior frontal gyrus
GFsd: superior part of the medial frontal gyrus
GOm: middle occipital gyrus
GOs: superior occipital gyrus
GPoC: postcentral gyrus
GPrC: precentral gyrus
GSM: supramarginal gyrus
IFS: inferior frontal sulcus
LPi: inferior parietal lobule
LPs: superior parietal lobule
M. Cing: middle cingulate gyrus
P. Cing: posterior cingulate gyrus
PoCS: postcentral sulcus
PrCS: precentral sulcus
PrCu: precuneus
SFS: superior frontal sulcus
SOS: superior occipital sulcus
Spl: splenium

z = 45 mm from the Anterior Commissure – Posterior Commissure Line

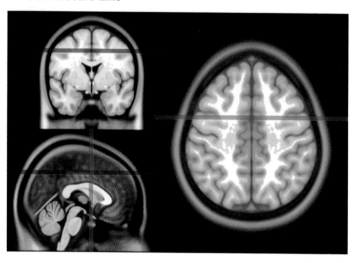

z = 52 mm from the Anterior Commissure – Posterior Commissure Line

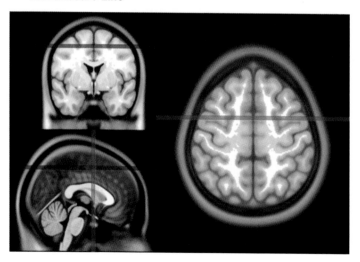

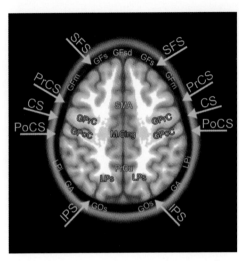

CS: central sulcus
GA: angular gyrus
GFm: middle frontal gyrus
GFs: superior frontal gyrus
GFsd: superior part of the medial frontal gyrus
GOs: superior occipital gyrus
GPoC: postcentral gyrus
GPrC: precentral gyrus
IPS: intraparietal sulcus
LPi: inferior parietal lobule
LPs: superior parietal lobule
M. Cing: middle cingulate gyrus
PCL: paracentral lobule
PoCS: postcentral sulcus
PrCS: precentral sulcus
PrCu: precuneus
SFS: superior frontal sulcus
SMA: supplementary motor area

PART
2

[Memo]

Cerebral Arterial Topography

Dong-Eog Kim, MD, PhD

Conventional Cartoon Maps vs.
New Supratentorial Probabilistic Maps: MRI & CT

Conventional Maps I

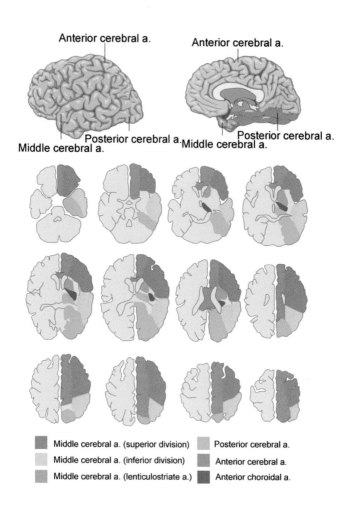

Anterior cerebral a.

Anterior cerebral a.

Posterior cerebral a.

Posterior cerebral a.

Middle cerebral a.

Middle cerebral a.

- ▉ Middle cerebral a. (superior division)
- ▉ Middle cerebral a. (inferior division)
- ▉ Middle cerebral a. (lenticulostriate a.)
- ▉ Posterior cerebral a.
- ▉ Anterior cerebral a.
- ▉ Anterior choroidal a.

Conventional Maps II

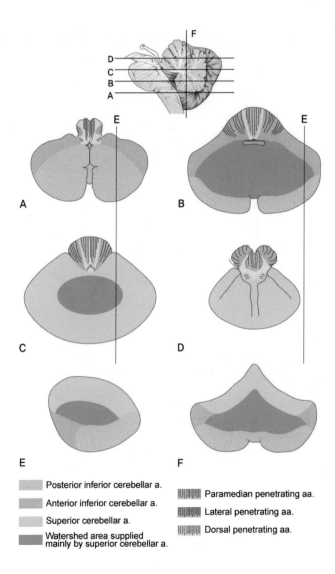

Posterior inferior cerebellar a.

Anterior inferior cerebellar a.

Superior cerebellar a.

Watershed area supplied mainly by superior cerebellar a.

Paramedian penetrating aa.

Lateral penetrating aa.

Dorsal penetrating aa.

(A) New Supratentorial Probabilistic Maps: MRI

(Updated from Dong-Eog Kim *et al.* Mapping the supratentorial cerebral arterial territories using 1160 large artery infarcts. *JAMA Neurology* 2019; 76:80.)

Figures

(1) Brain MRI Templates Used for Territorial Mapping

(2) Infarct Frequency MRI Maps with Color Blending for Interterritorial Overlap Areas

(3) Infarct Frequency MRI Maps without Overlap Areas

(4) Certainty Index (CI) MRI Maps for the Anterior Cerebral Artery

(5) Certainty Index (CI) MRI Maps for the Middle Cerebral Artery

(6) Certainty Index (CI) MRI Maps for the Posterior Cerebral Artery

(7) Interterritorial Border Zone MRI Maps

(8) Interterritorial Border Line MRI Maps

Table

Table 1. Mean Certainty Index (%) for a Brain Region to be Designated as a Vascular Territory.

Please note that undetermined regions in the maps include the areas where infarcts are infrequently observed, such as orbitofrontal regions and frontal tips, both of which are known to be the anterior cerebral artery territory.

(1) Brain MRI Templates Used for Territorial Mapping

MNI ICBM 152 T1 template: z = -16, -10, -4, 2, 9, 15, 21, 27, 33, 39, 45, and 52 mm from the anterior commissure – posterior commissure line. (See also pages 4 – 15 for slice information.)

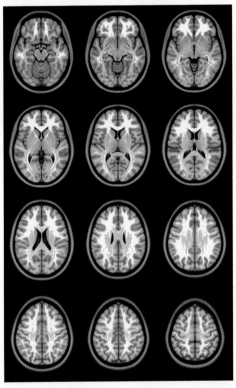

1. VS Fonov, AC Evans, K Botteron, *et al.* Unbiased average age-appropriate atlases for pediatric studies. *NeuroImage* 2011; 54: 313 – 327. ISSN 1053 – 8119, DOI: 10.1016/j. neuroimage.2010.07.033.

2. VS Fonov, AC Evans, RC McKinstry, *et al.* Unbiased nonlinear average age-appropriate brain templates from birth to adulthood. *NeuroImage* 2009; 47:S102. Organization for Human Brain Mapping 2009 Annual Meeting. DOI: http://dx.doi.org/10.1016/ S1053-8119(09)70884-5.

(2) Infarct Frequency MRI Maps with Color Blending for Interterritorial Overlap Areas: green, red, and blue for anterior, middle, and posterior cerebral artery, respectively.

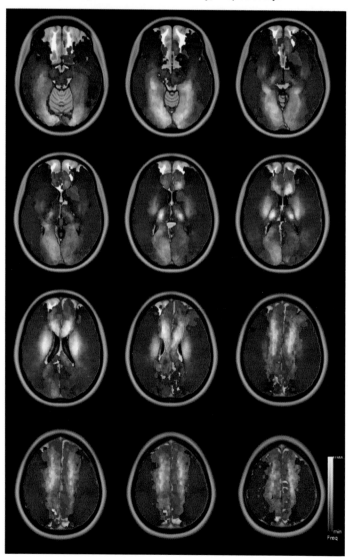

(Transparent version)

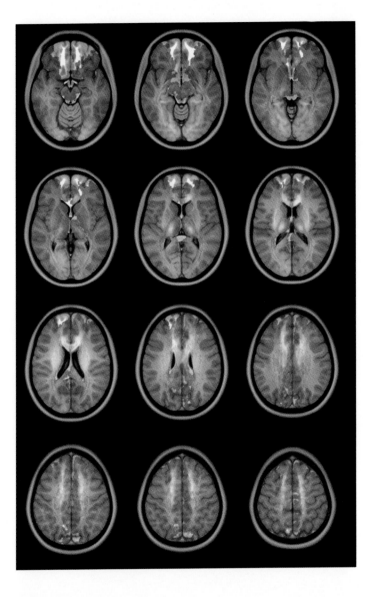

(3) Infarct Frequency MRI Maps Allocating Each Voxel in Interterritorial Overlap Areas as the Territory of a Cerebral Artery Associated With the Highest Infarct Frequency on the Voxel: green, red, and blue for anterior, middle, and posterior cerebral artery, respectively.

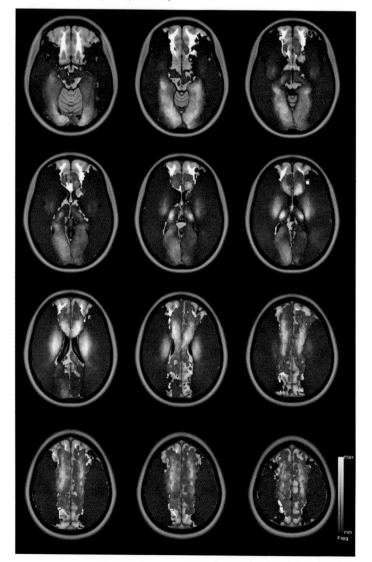

(Transparent version)

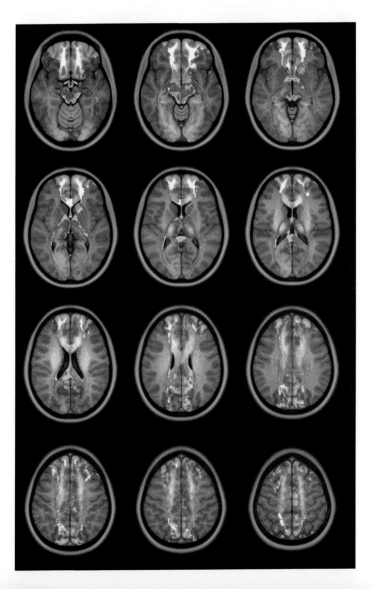

(4) Certainty Index (CI) MRI Maps for the Anterior Cerebral Artery: CI reflects the likelihood of a voxel being a member of a specific vascular territory vs. the other territories.

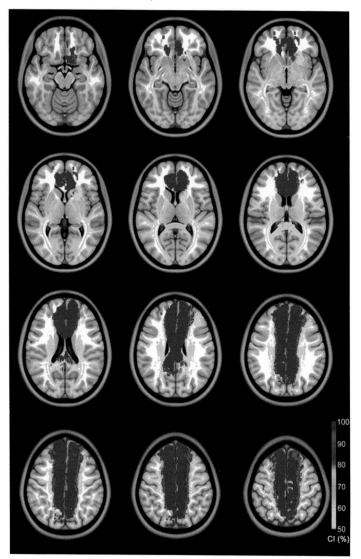

(Transparent version)

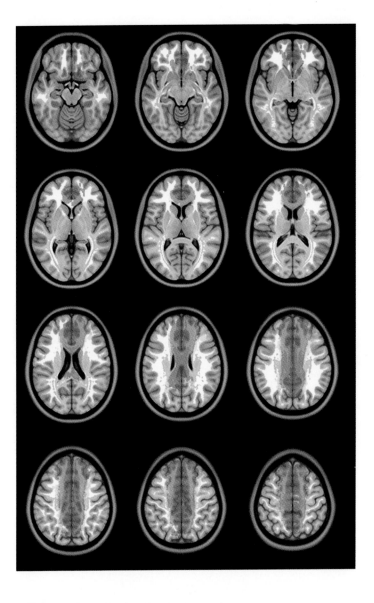

(5) Certainty Index (CI) MRI Maps for the Middle Cerebral Artery:
CI reflects the likelihood of a voxel being a member of a specific vascular territory vs. the other territories.

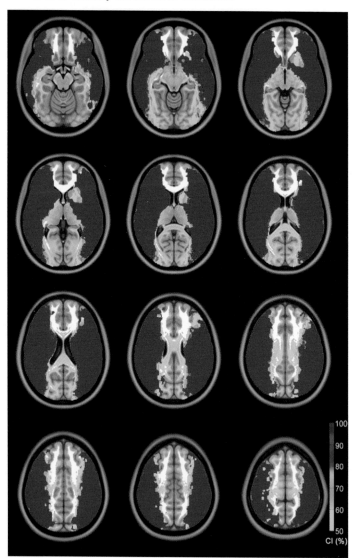

(Transparent version)

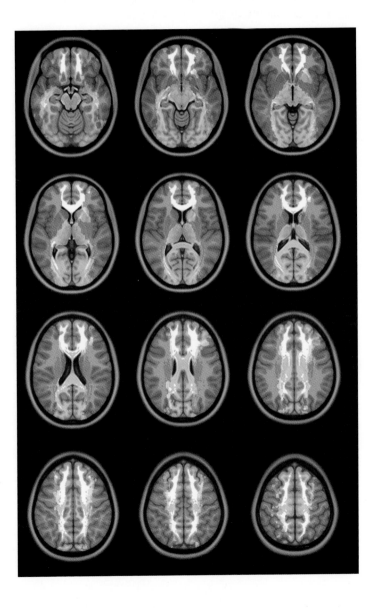

(6) Certainty Index (CI) MRI Maps for the Posterior Cerebral Artery: CI reflects the likelihood of a voxel being a member of a specific vascular territory vs. the other territories.

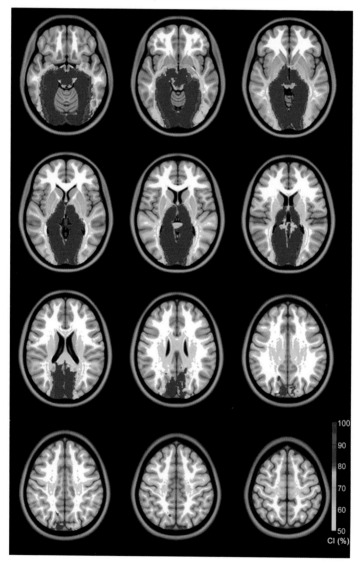

(Transparent version)

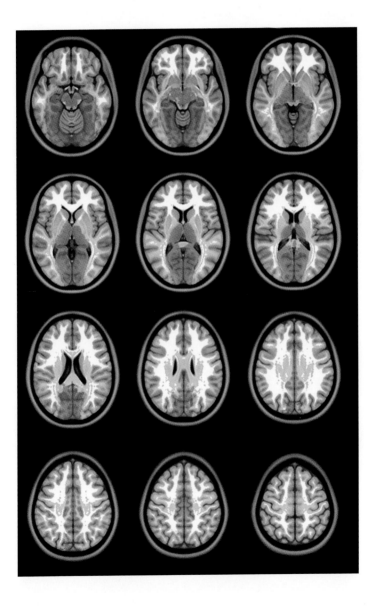

(7) Interterritorial Border Zone MRI Maps: vascular territorial
overlaps depicted, as derived from the infarct frequency maps on
page 24. (ACA = anterior cerebral artery; MCA = middle cerebral
artery; PCA = posterior cerebral artery.)

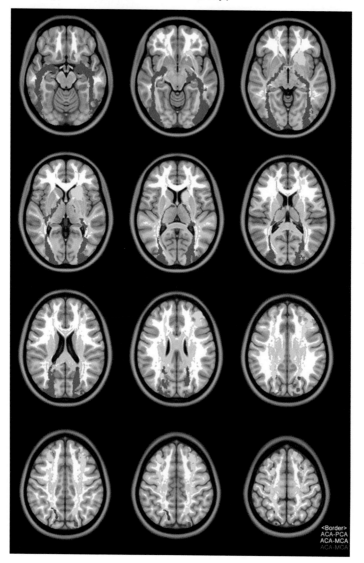

(Transparent version)

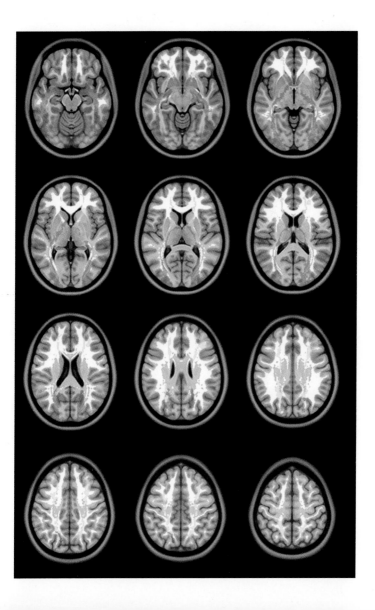

(8) Interterritorial Border Line MRI Maps: certainty Index (CI) difference MRI maps generated by forcing a choice for each voxel to belong to only 1 parent vessel. (See CI maps in pages 28 – 33.)

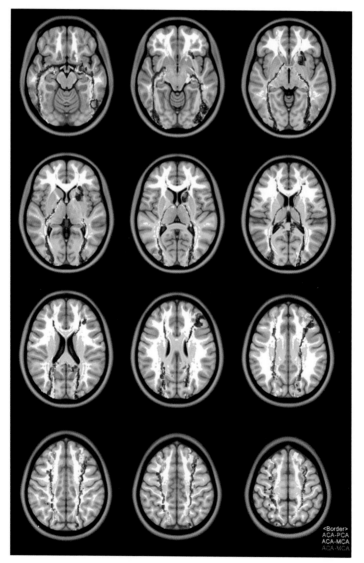

<Border>
ACA-PCA
ACA-MCA
ACA-MCA

(Transparent version)

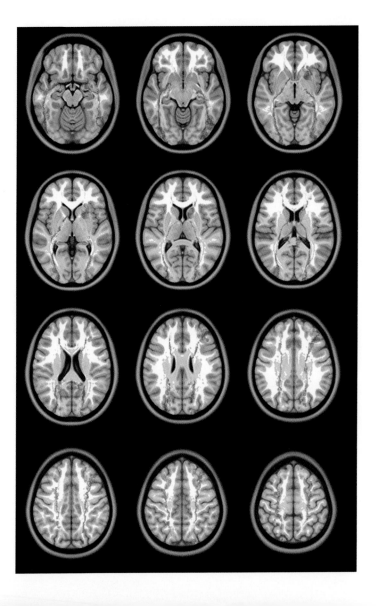

Table 1. Mean Certainty Index (%) for a Brain Region to Be Designated as a Vascular Territory. (See pages 4 – 15 for slice information (z from AC-PC line) and page 45 for abbreviations.)

z* from AC-PC (mm)	Art.	Frontal				
		GFs	GFso	GFm	GFmo	GFio
-16	ACA		3.0		0.0	0.0
	MCA		13.4		39.1	92.4
	PCA		<0.1		<0.1	<0.1
-10	ACA		1.1		1.9	1.5
	MCA		2.4		79.2	95.4
	PCA		<0.1		<0.1	<0.1
-4	ACA		13.9	<0.1		<0.1
	MCA		35.5	95.4		97.0
	PCA		<0.1	<0.1		<0.1
2	ACA	12.4		0.6		
	MCA	21.7		89.0		
	PCA	<0.1		<0.1		
9	ACA	1.6		<0.1		
	MCA	49.8		95.3		
	PCA	<0.1		<0.1		
15	ACA	5.8		1.5		
	MCA	40.6		94.9		
	PCA	<0.1		<0.1		
21	ACA	34.7		6.9		
	MCA	9.7		86.7		
	PCA	<0.1		<0.1		
27	ACA	39.0		31.4		
	MCA	19.8		65.2		
	PCA	<0.1		<0.1		
33	ACA	74.6		27.0		
	MCA	18.4		71.2		
	PCA	<0.1		<0.1		
39	ACA	76.6		15.0		
	MCA	13.7		82.4		
	PCA	<0.1		<0.1		
45	ACA	93.5		31.8		
	MCA	4.0		66.0		
	PCA	<0.1		<0.1		
52	ACA	85.1		17.7		
	MCA	9.8		76.9		
	PCA	<0.1		<0.1		
All	ACA	55.2	4.9	14.4	0.9	0.6
	MCA	19.3	15.4	81.2	58.1	94.8
	PCA	<0.1	<0.1	<0.1	<0.1	<0.1

GFiop	GFi	GFdo	GFsd	Rectus	SMA	GPrC
				11.4		
				0.2		
				<0.1		
		14.0				
		<0.1				
		<0.1				
		5.9				
		<0.1				
		<0.1				
<0.1	<0.1		0.6			
97.0	96.9		<0.1			
<0.1	<0.1		<0.1			
<0.1	<0.1		37.0			
97.0	97.0		0.1			
<0.1	<0.1		<0.1			
<0.1	<0.1		53.3			<0.1
97.0	97.0		1.2			97.0
<0.1	<0.1		<0.1			<0.1
<0.1	<0.1		80.0			<0.1
96.5	97.0		1.1			97.0
<0.1	<0.1		<0.1			<0.1
<0.1	8.1		79.4			<0.1
97.0	89.5		0.1			97.0
<0.1	<0.1		<0.1			<0.1
6.0			82.7			0.6
91.5			<0.1			96.5
<0.1			<0.1			<0.1
			88.5			2.3
			0.1			95.0
			<0.1			<0.1
			89.7		91.5	17.4
			0.1		0.1	80.4
			<0.1		<0.1	<0.1
			72.2		89.9	12.3
			0.6		0.1	85.3
			<0.1		<0.1	<0.1
1.2	1.3	10.7	68.3	11.4	90.4	7.1
95.8	95.8	<0.1	0.3	0.2	0.1	90.3
<0.1	<0.1	<0.1	<0.1	<0.1	<0.1	<0.1

Table 1 (*continued*): Mean Certainty Index (%) for Various Regions of Interest (ROIs) to be Designated as a Vascular Territory.

z* from AC-PC (mm)	Art.	Temporal				
		GTps	GTs	GTm	GTi	GH
-16	ACA	<0.1	<0.1	<0.1	<0.1	
	MCA	83.3	90.2	86.9	81.2	
	PCA	<0.1	6.1	9.2	16.2	
-10	ACA	<0.1	<0.1	<0.1	<0.1	
	MCA	86.7	95.5	95.3	85.0	
	PCA	<0.1	1.8	2.0	13.0	
-4	ACA	<0.1	<0.1	<0.1		
	MCA	96.7	97.0	97.0		
	PCA	<0.1	<0.1	0.1		
2	ACA		<0.1	<0.1		
	MCA		96.9	97.0		
	PCA		0.1	<0.1		
9	ACA		<0.1	<0.1		<0.1
	MCA		97.0	96.9		95.9
	PCA		<0.1	0.1		0.4
15	ACA		<0.1	<0.1		
	MCA		96.5	97.0		
	PCA		<0.1	<0.1		
21	ACA		<0.1	<0.1		
	MCA		97.0	97.0		
	PCA		<0.1	<0.1		
27	ACA					
	MCA					
	PCA					
33	ACA					
	MCA					
	PCA					
39	ACA					
	MCA					
	PCA					
45	ACA					
	MCA					
	PCA					
52	ACA					
	MCA					
	PCA					
All	ACA	<0.1	<0.1	<0.1	<0.1	<0.1
	MCA	90.5	96.0	95.1	82.5	95.9
	PCA	<0.1	0.9	1.8	15.1	0.4

			Parietal				
GpH	**Am**	**LPs**	**LPi**	**GSM**	**GA**	**PrCu**	**GPoC**
<0.1	<0.1						
0.1	46.9						
95.6	52.8						
<0.1							
0.7							
92.5							
<0.1							
0.3							
97.0							
				<0.1		0.8	<0.1
				97.0		<0.1	**97.0**
				<0.1		**80.9**	<0.1
				<0.1		5.9	<0.1
				97.0		<0.1	**97.0**
				<0.1		66.7	<0.1
				<0.1	<0.1	34.9	<0.1
				97.0	**97.0**	1.0	**97.0**
				<0.1	<0.1	47.9	<0.1
				<0.1	<0.1	**84.6**	<0.1
				97.0	**97.0**	2.8	**97.0**
				<0.1	<0.1	1.7	<0.1
		2.3	0.4	<0.1	0.1	75.0	<0.1
		94.9	**96.5**	**97.0**	**96.9**	2.0	**97.0**
		<0.1	<0.1	<0.1	<0.1	3.5	<0.1
		22.4	0.9		<0.1	76.8	2.3
		52.3	**96.1**		**97.0**	0.7	**94.9**
		2.4	<0.1		<0.1	2.7	<0.1
		11.6	2.7		2.6	84.2	9.5
		81.0	**94.2**		**91.9**	1.1	**88.0**
		0.7	<0.1		<0.1	0.5	<0.1
<0.1	<0.1	14.7	1.3	<0.1	0.1	61.0	2.2
0.4	46.9	72.0	**95.6**	**97.0**	**96.8**	1.2	**95.0**
94.7	52.8	1.2	<0.1	<0.1	<0.1	20.3	<0.1

Table 1 (*continued*)

z* from AC-PC (mm)	Art.	Occipital				
		GOs	GOm	GOi	Cal	Cu
-16	ACA			<0.1	<0.1	
	MCA			52.6	0.1	
	PCA			42.5	55.0	
-10	ACA			<0.1	<0.1	
	MCA			42.7	1.9	
	PCA			57.1	**94.2**	
-4	ACA		<0.1	<0.1	<0.1	
	MCA		69.6	**92.4**	7.9	
	PCA		30.0	5.5	**88.5**	
2	ACA		<0.1		<0.1	
	MCA		76.0		1.7	
	PCA		22.4		**95.9**	
9	ACA		<0.1		<0.1	
	MCA		69.3		0.1	
	PCA		29.2		**93.1**	
15	ACA	<0.1	<0.1		<0.1	<0.1
	MCA	27.1	74.9		0.2	2.0
	PCA	72.0	23.4		**95.3**	**92.1**
21	ACA	<0.1	<0.1		<0.1	1.0
	MCA	47.0	**93.5**		0.4	2.1
	PCA	52.2	3.9		**96.7**	**92.3**
27	ACA	0.7	<0.1			2.1
	MCA	59.9	**95.7**			6.2
	PCA	36.8	1.4			70.3
33	ACA	2.5	<0.1			10.7
	MCA	86.8	**97.0**			15.1
	PCA	8.2	<0.1			49.9
39	ACA	12.6	<0.1			8.3
	MCA	62.3	**97.0**			13.1
	PCA	17.2	<0.1			27.0
45	ACA	3.9				
	MCA	69.5				
	PCA	14.4				
52	ACA					
	MCA					
	PCA					
All	ACA	3.9	<0.1	<0.1	<0.1	3.4
	MCA	62.0	79.8	57.9	2.2	6.3
	PCA	30.0	18.3	40.5	**90.9**	72.8

	Cingulate		Others				
A. Cing	M. Cing	P. Cing	Ins	GF	GL	PCL	Rop.
				<0.1	<0.1		
				6.2	3.4		
				90.6	91.5		
47.0			<0.1	<0.1	<0.1		
<0.1			96.9	2.4	<0.1		
<0.1			0.2	95.8	91.3		
75.0			2.0		<0.1		
<0.1			95.2		0.1		
<0.1			<0.1		96.2		
79.4			2.6		<0.1		<0.1
<0.1			94.6		<0.1		97.0
<0.1			<0.1		92.4		<0.1
92.9			<0.1		<0.1		<0.1
0.1			97.0		<0.1		96.5
<0.1			<0.1		84.2		<0.1
95.6			<0.1				<0.1
<0.1			97.0				97.0
<0.1			<0.1				<0.1
93.2		27.7					<0.1
<0.1		<0.1					97.0
<0.1		41.4					<0.1
90.6		44.0					
0.1		<0.1					
<0.1		4.1					
	91.3	91.2					
	<0.1	<0.1					
	<0.1	<0.1					
	90.9						
	0.3						
	<0.1						
	92.0						
	0.1						
	<0.1						
						74.2	
						<0.1	
						<0.1	
84.3	91.3	57.2	1.3	<0.1	<0.1	74.2	<0.1
<0.1	0.1	<0.1	95.8	5.2	0.8	<0.1	96.9
<0.1	<0.1	12.2	<0.1	91.9	93.0	<0.1	<0.1

Table 1 (*continued*)

z* from AC-PC (mm)	Art.	Thalamostriatal Region			
		Thal	Ca	GP	Put
-16	ACA				
	MCA				
	PCA				
-10	ACA		5.0		3.0
	MCA		48.7		90.3
	PCA		<0.1		0.9
-4	ACA		27.5	<0.1	9.9
	MCA		52.4	97.0	87.2
	PCA		3.6	<0.1	0.8
2	ACA	<0.1	23.7	6.5	14.7
	MCA	<0.1	68.2	90.9	83.5
	PCA	94.0	1.3	<0.1	<0.1
9	ACA	<0.1	20.8		3.3
	MCA	<0.1	74.4		94.2
	PCA	85.3	<0.1		<0.1
15	ACA	<0.1	8.5		
	MCA	0.5	85.1		
	PCA	92.2	0.3		
21	ACA		5.3		
	MCA		71.9		
	PCA		<0.1		
27	ACA				
	MCA				
	PCA				
33	ACA				
	MCA				
	PCA				
39	ACA				
	MCA				
	PCA				
45	ACA				
	MCA				
	PCA				
52	ACA				
	MCA				
	PCA				
All	ACA	<0.1	16.0	3.0	7.8
	MCA	0.1	68.1	94.2	89.0
	PCA	91.1	0.9	<0.1	0.4

Values higher than 50 are colored, and values higher than 80 are in bold characters.

A 'CI' reflects the likelihood of a voxel being a member of a specific vascular territory, calculated as the ratio of frequency of infarction related to the relevant parent vessel divided by the sum of infarct frequencies for all vascular territories in that voxel.

Abbreviations: AC – PC, anterior commissure – posterior commissure; Art, artery; A, anterior; M, middle; P, posterior; ACA, anterior cerebral artery; MCA, middle cerebral artery; PCA, posterior cerebral artery.

A.Cing	Anterior cingulate gyrus	GpH	Parahippocampal gyrus
Am	Amygdala	GPoC	Postcentral gyrus
Ca	Caudate	GPrC	Precentral gyrus
Cal	Calcarine gyrus	GSM	Supramarginal gyrus
Cu	Cuneus	GTi	Inferior temporal gyrus
GA	Angular gyrus	GTm	Middle temporal gyrus
GF	fusiform gyrus	GTps	Superior temporo-polar gyrus
GFdo	Orbital part of the medial frontal gyrus	GTs	Superior temporal gyrus
GFi	Inferior frontal gyrus	Ins	Insula
GFio	Orbital part of the inferior frontal gyrus	LPi	Inferior parietal lobule
GFiop	Opercular part of the inferior frontal gyrus	LPs	Superior parietal lobule
GFm	Middle frontal gyrus	M.Cing	Middle cingulate gyrus
GFmo	Orbital part of the middle frontal gyrus	Olf	Olfactory gyrus
GFs	Superior frontal gyrus	P.Cing	Posterior cingulate gyrus
GFsd	Superior part of the medial frontal gyrus	PCL	Paracentral lobule
GFso	Orbital part of the superior frontal gyrus	PrCu	Precentral sulcus
GH	Heschl gyrus	Put	Putamen
GL	Lingual gyrus	Rectus	Gyrus rectus
GOi	Inferior occipital gyrus	Rop	Rolandic operculum
GOm	Middle occipital gyrus	SMA	Supplementary motor area
GOs	Superior occipital gyrus	Spl	Splenium
GP	Globus pallidus	Thal	Thalamus

(B) New Supratentorial Probabilistic Maps: CT

from Dong-Eog Kim *et al.* Supratentorial cerebral arterial territories for computed tomograms: a mapping study in 1160 large artery infarcts. *Scientific Reports;* 2019 9:11708.

Figures

(1) Brain CT Templates used for Territorial Mapping

(2) Infarct Frequency CT Maps with Color Blending for Interterritorial Overlap Areas

(3) Infarct Frequency CT Maps without Overlap Areas

(4) Certainty Index (CI) CT Maps for the Anterior Cerebral Artery

(5) Certainty Index (CI) CT Maps for the Middle Cerebral Artery

(6) Certainty Index (CI) CT Maps for the Posterior Cerebral Artery

(7) Interterritorial Border Zone CT Maps

(8) Interterritorial Border Line CT Maps

Please note that undetermined regions in the maps include the areas where infarcts are infrequently observed, such as the orbitofrontal regions and frontal tips, both of which are known to be the anterior cerebral artery territory.

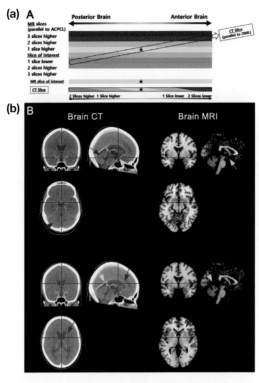

Different slice angles for axial MR vs. CT images. (a) The anterior-posterior commissure line (ACPCL) and orbitomeatal line (OML) for the image slicing of respectively MRI and CT are not parallel. Because of the pitch angle difference (9°) between the imaging reference lines, the anterior and posterior portions of the axial CT image is respectively about –10 mm lower and higher in the z-axis, with the central portion overlapping around the rotation point, centered on the MR slice of interest (asterisks). Here, 10-mm difference corresponds to about 2-slice difference, because the slice thicknesses of MRI and CT are respectively 6 mm and 5 mm. **(b)** Anatomical matching of the anterior portions in the MR and CT images (yellow arrows in the upper panel figures) causes a mismatching of the posterior portions (red arrows in the upper panel figures), and vice versa (yellow and red arrows in the lower panel figures).

(1) Brain CT Templates Used for Territorial Mapping: prepared by realigning the originally anterior/posterior commissure line-aligned stroke-control CT template (Rorden, C. *et al. Neuroimage*; 2019; 61:957 – 965) so that they become parallel to the orbitomeatal line.

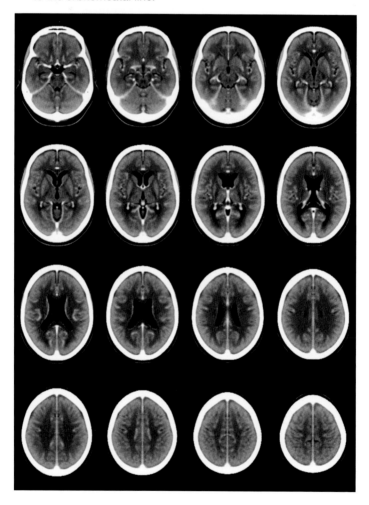

(2) Infarct Frequency CT Maps with Color Blending for Interterritorial Overlap Areas: green, red, and blue for anterior, middle, and posterior cerebral artery, respectively.

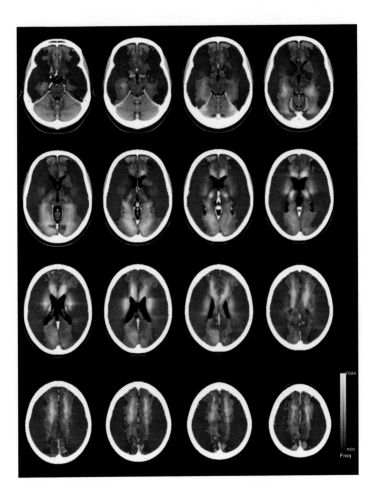

(3) Infarct Frequency CT Maps Allocating Each Voxel in Interterritorial Overlap Areas as the Territory of a Cerebral Artery associated with the Highest Infarct Frequency on the Voxel: green, red, and blue for anterior, middle, and posterior cerebral artery, respectively.

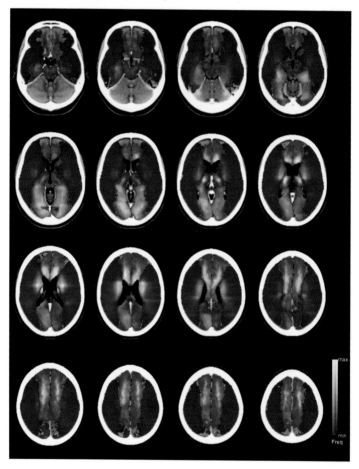

(4) Certainty Index (CI) CT Maps for the Anterior Cerebral Artery:
CI reflects the likelihood of a voxel being a member of a specific vascular territory vs. the other territories.

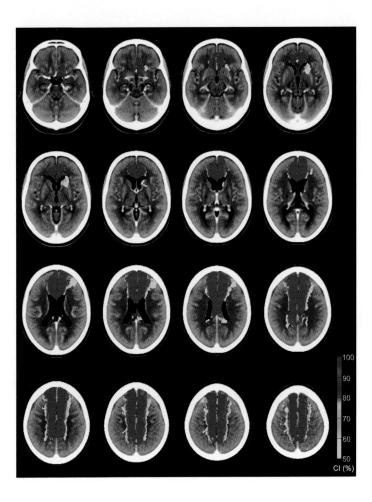

(5) Certainty Index (CI) CT Maps for the Middle Cerebral Artery: CI reflects the likelihood of a voxel being a member of a specific vascular territory vs. the other territories.

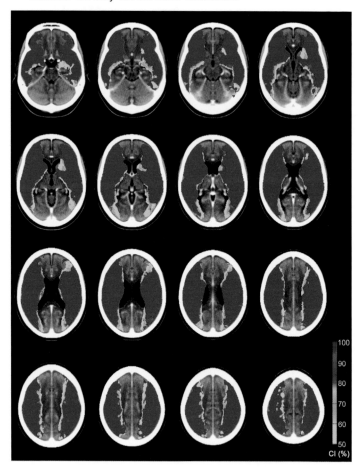

(6) Certainty Index (CI) CT Maps for the Posterior Cerebral Artery: CI reflects the likelihood of a voxel being a member of a specific vascular territory vs. the other territories.

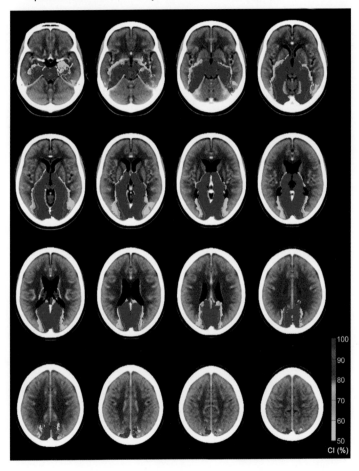

(7) Interterritorial Border Zone CT Maps: vascular territorial overlaps depicted, as derived from the infarct frequency maps on page 49. (ACA = anterior cerebral artery; MCA = middle cerebral artery; PCA = posterior cerebral artery.)

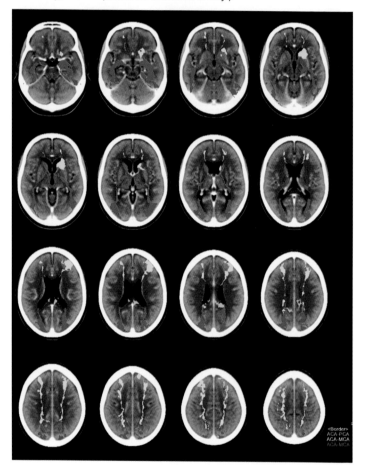

(8) Interterritorial Border Line CT Maps: Certainty Index (CI) difference MRI maps generated by forcing a choice for each Voxel to belong to only 1 parent vessel. (See CI Maps on pages 51 – 53.)

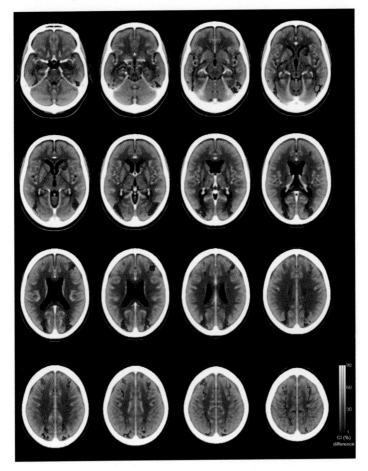

PART
3

[Memo]

Cerebral Arterial Anatomy and Topography for Coronal Sections

Jung E Park, MD; Da-Hye Heo, BS;
Dong-Eog Kim, MD, PhD

Please note that undetermined regions in the maps include the areas where infarcts are infrequently observed, such as the orbitofrontal regions and frontal tips, both of which are known to be the anterior cerebral artery territory.

Coronal Brain MRI Templates Used for Territorial Mapping

MNI ICBM 152 T1 template: y = 60, 55, 50, 45, 40, 35, 30, 25, 20, 15, 10, 5, 0, -5, -10, -15, -20, -25, -30, -35, -40, -45, -50, -55, -60, -65, -70, -75, -80 mm from the origin (anterior commissure).

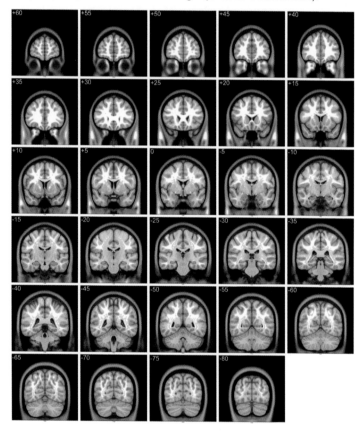

1. VS Fonov, AC Evans, K Botteron, CR Almli, RC McKinstry, DL Collins and BDCG. Unbiased average age-appropriate atlases for pediatric studies. *NeuroImage* 2011; 54: 313-327. ISSN 1053–8119, DOI: 10.1016/j.neuroimage.2010.07.033.

2. VS Fonov, AC Evans, RC McKinstry, CR Almli and DL Collins. Unbiased nonlinear average age-appropriate brain templates from birth to adulthood. *NeuroImage* 2009; 47: S102. Organization for Human Brain Mapping 2009 Annual Meeting, DOI: http://dx.doi.org/10.1016/S1053-8119(09)70884-5.

Abbreviations

A.Cing	Anterior cingulate gyrus	GP	Globus pallidus
Am	Amygdala	GpH	Parahippocampal gyrus
Ca	Caudate	GPoC	Postcentral gyrus
Cal	Calcarine gyrus	GPrC	Precentral gyrus
Cu	Cuneus	GSM	Supramarginal gyrus
GA	Angular gyrus	GTi	Inferior temporal gyrus
GF	Fusiform gyrus	GTm	Middle temporal gyrus
GFdo	Orbital part of the medial frontal gyrus	GTps	Superior temporo-polar gyrus
GFi	Inferior frontal gyrus	GTs	Superior temporal gyrus
GFio	Orbital part of the inferior frontal gyrus	Ins	Insula
GFiop	Opercular part of the inferior frontal gyrus	LPi	Inferior parietal lobule
GFm	Middle frontal gyrus	LPs	Superior parietal lobule
GFmo	Orbital part of the middle frontal gyrus	M.Cing	Middle cingulate gyrus
GFs	Superior frontal gyrus	P.Cing	Posterior cingulate gyrus
GFsd	Superior part of the medial frontal gyrus	PCL	Paracentral lobule
GFso	Orbital part of the superior frontal gyrus	PrCu	Precentral sulcus
GH	Heschl gyrus	Put	Putamen
GL	Lingual gyrus	Rectus	Gyrus rectus
GOi	Inferior occipital gyrus	Rop	Rolandic operculum
GOm	Middle occipital gyrus	SMA	Supplementary motor area
GOs	Superior occipital gyrus	Thal	Thalamus

Certainty Index (CI) Coronal (y = +60) MRI Maps: CI Reflects the Likelihood of a Voxel being a Member of a Specific Vascular Territory vs. the Other Territories.

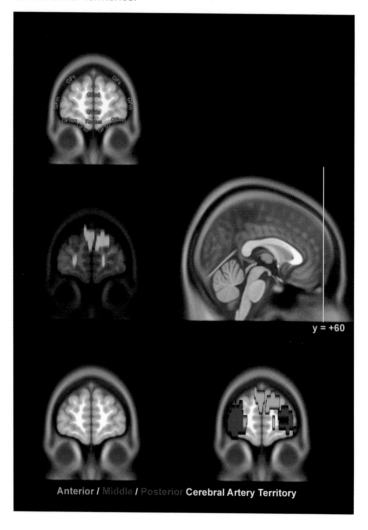

Anterior / Middle / Posterior **Cerebral Artery Territory**

Certainty Index (CI) Coronal (y = +55) MRI Maps: CI Reflects the Likelihood of a Voxel being a Member of a Specific Vascular Territory vs. the Other Territories.

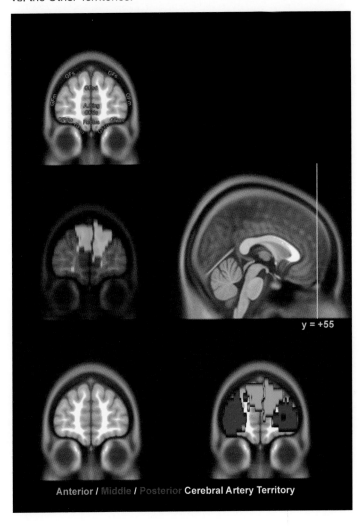

Anterior / Middle / Posterior Cerebral Artery Territory

Certainty Index (CI) Coronal (y = +50) MRI Maps: CI Reflects the Likelihood of a Voxel being a Member of a Specific Vascular Territory vs. the Other Territories.

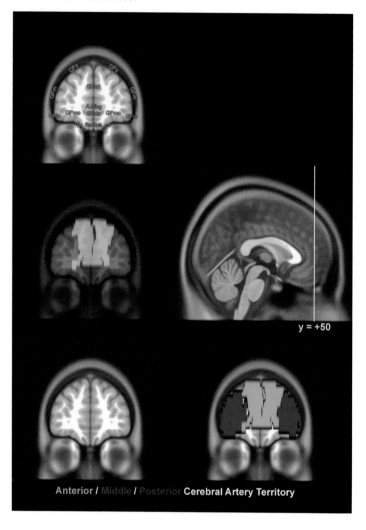

Anterior / Middle / Posterior **Cerebral Artery Territory**

Certainty Index (CI) Coronal (y = +45) MRI Maps: CI Reflects the Likelihood of a Voxel being a Member of a Specific Vascular Territory vs. the Other Territories.

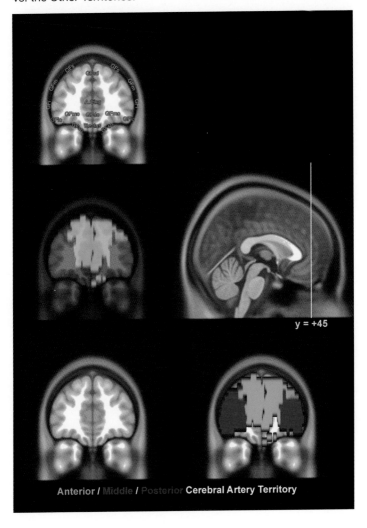

Anterior / Middle / Posterior **Cerebral Artery Territory**

Certainty Index (CI) Coronal (y = +40) MRI Maps: CI Reflects the Likelihood of a Voxel being a Member of a Specific Vascular Territory vs. the Other Territories.

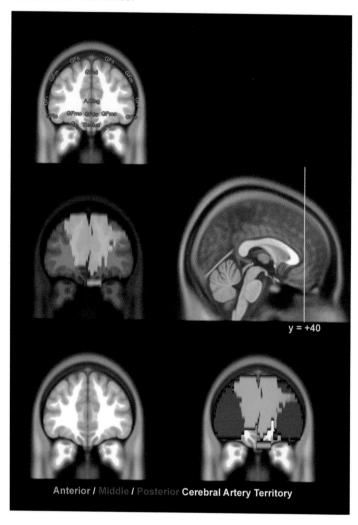

Anterior / Middle / Posterior Cerebral Artery Territory

Certainty Index (CI) Coronal (y = +35) MRI Maps: CI Reflects the Likelihood of a Voxel being a Member of a Specific Vascular Territory vs. the Other Territories.

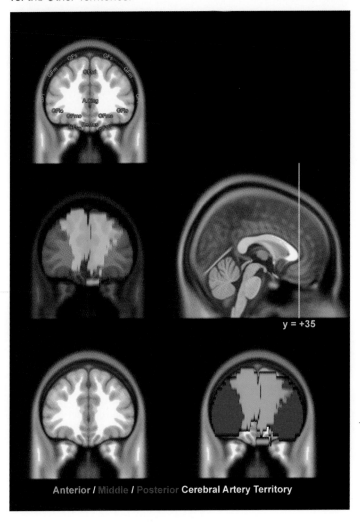

Anterior / Middle / Posterior **Cerebral Artery Territory**

Certainty Index (CI) Coronal (y = +30) MRI Maps: CI Reflects the Likelihood of a Voxel being a Member of a Specific Vascular Territory vs. the Other Territories.

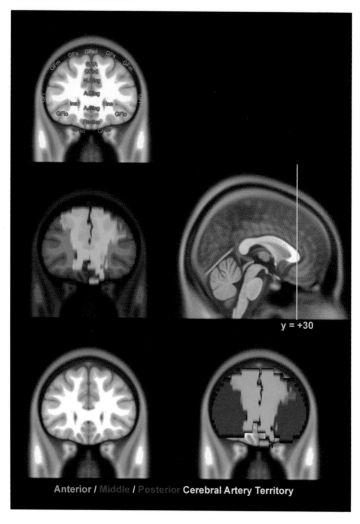

Anterior / Middle / Posterior Cerebral Artery Territory

Certainty Index (CI) Coronal (y = +25) MRI Maps: CI Reflects the Likelihood of a Voxel being a Member of a Specific Vascular Territory vs. the Other Territories.

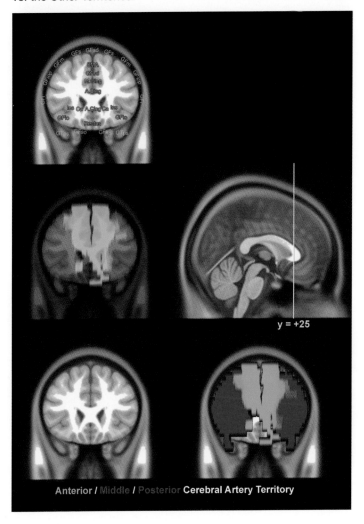

Anterior / Middle **/** Posterior **Cerebral Artery Territory**

Certainty Index (CI) Coronal (y = +20) MRI Maps; CI Reflects the Likelihood of a Voxel being a Member of a Specific Vascular Territory vs. the Other Territories.

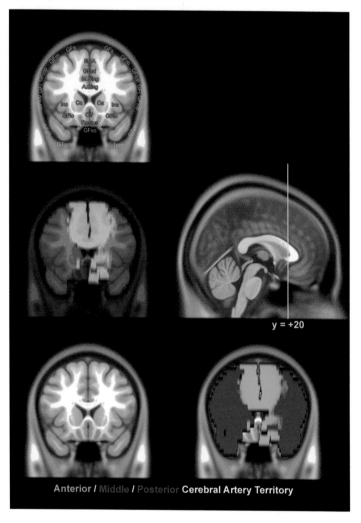

Anterior / Middle / Posterior **Cerebral Artery Territory**

Certainty Index (CI) Coronal (y = +15) MRI Maps; CI Reflects the Likelihood of a Voxel being a Member of a Specific Vascular Territory vs. the Other Territories.

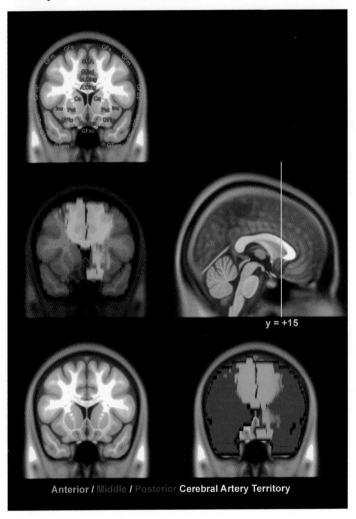

Anterior / Middle / Posterior **Cerebral Artery Territory**

Certainty Index (CI) Coronal (y = +10) MRI Maps: CI Reflects the Likelihood of a Voxel being a Member of a Specific Vascular Territory vs. the Other Territories.

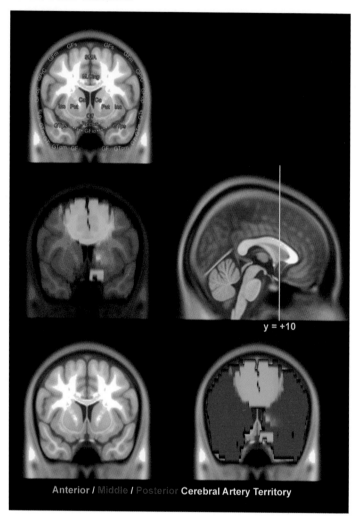

Anterior / Middle / Posterior **Cerebral Artery Territory**

Certainty Index (CI) Coronal (y = +5) MRI Maps: CI Reflects the Likelihood of a Voxel being a Member of a Specific Vascular Territory vs. the Other Territories.

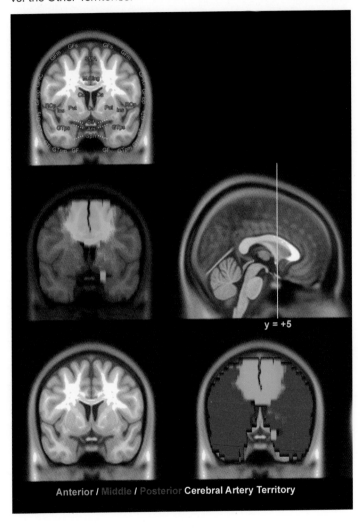

Anterior / Middle / Posterior **Cerebral Artery Territory**

Certainty Index (CI) Coronal (y = 0) MRI Maps: CI Reflects the Likelihood of a Voxel being a Member of a Specific Vascular Territory vs. the Other Territories.

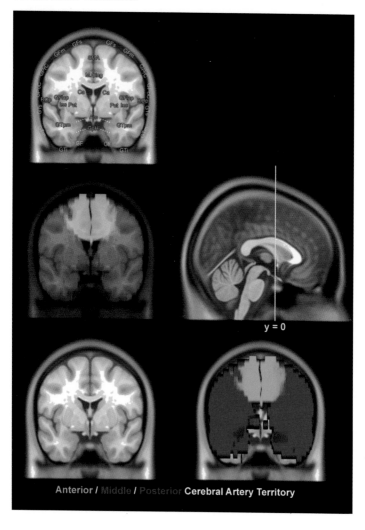

Anterior / Middle / Posterior Cerebral Artery Territory

Certainty Index (CI) Coronal (y = -5) MRI Maps: CI Reflects the Likelihood of a Voxel being a Member of a Specific Vascular Territory vs. the Other Territories.

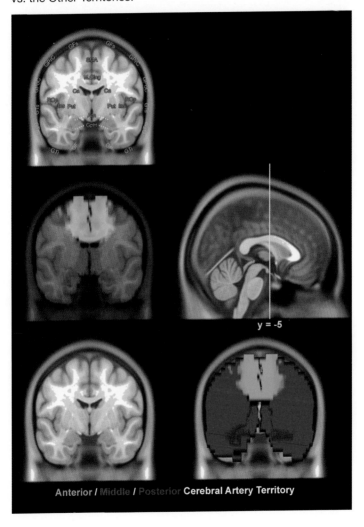

Anterior / Middle / Posterior Cerebral Artery Territory

Certainty Index (CI) Coronal (y = -10) MRI Maps: CI Reflects the Likelihood of a Voxel being a Member of a Specific Vascular Territory vs. the Other Territories.

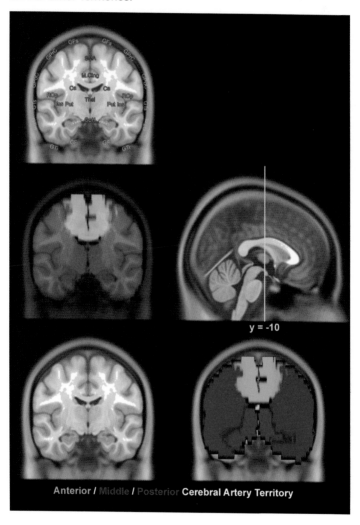

Anterior / Middle / Posterior Cerebral Artery Territory

Certainty Index (CI) Coronal (y = -15) MRI Maps: CI Reflects the Likelihood of a Voxel being a Member of a Specific Vascular Territory vs. the Other Territories.

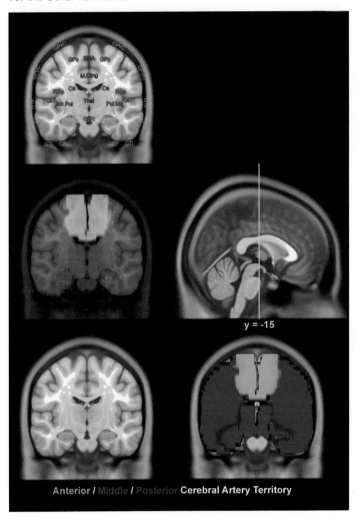

Anterior / Middle / Posterior **Cerebral Artery Territory**

Certainty Index (CI) Coronal (y = -20) MRI Maps: CI Reflects the Likelihood of a Voxel being a Member of a Specific Vascular Territory vs. the Other Territories.

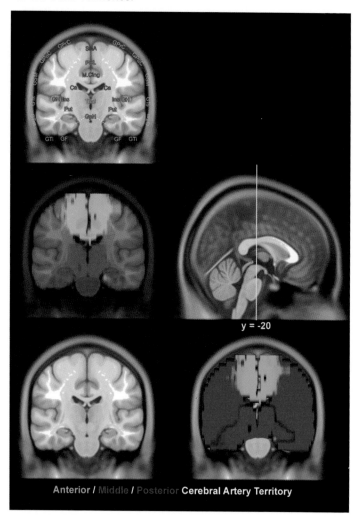

Anterior / Middle / Posterior Cerebral Artery Territory

Certainty Index (CI) Coronal (y = -25) MRI Maps: CI Reflects the Likelihood of a Voxel being a Member of a Specific Vascular Territory vs. the Other Territories.

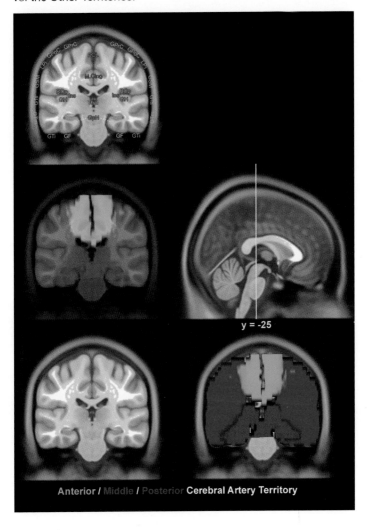

Anterior / Middle / Posterior Cerebral Artery Territory

Certainty Index (CI) Coronal (y = -30) MRI Maps: CI Reflects the Likelihood of a Voxel being a Member of a Specific Vascular Territory vs. the Other Territories.

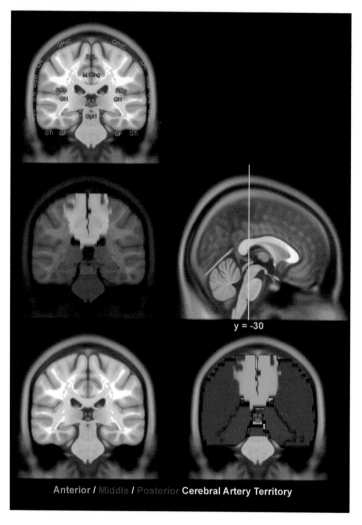

Anterior / Middle / Posterior Cerebral Artery Territory

Certainty Index (CI) Coronal (y = -35) MRI Maps: CI Reflects the Likelihood of a Voxel being a Member of a Specific Vascular Territory vs. the Other Territories.

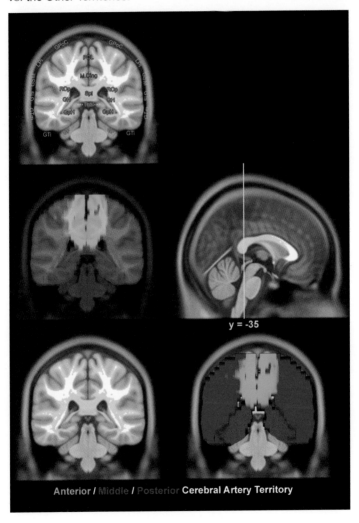

Anterior / Middle / Posterior **Cerebral Artery Territory**

Certainty Index (CI) Coronal (y = -40) MRI Maps: CI Reflects the Likelihood of a Voxel being a Member of a Specific Vascular Territory vs. the Other Territories.

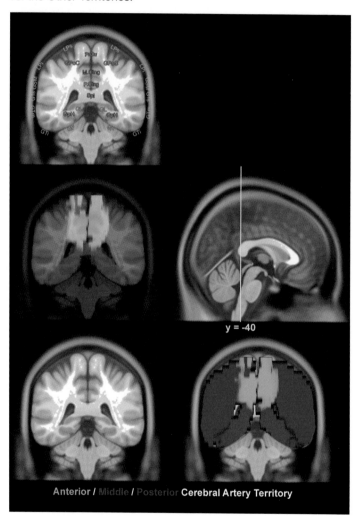

Anterior / Middle / Posterior **Cerebral Artery Territory**

Certainty Index (CI) Coronal (y = -45) MRI Maps: CI Reflects the Likelihood of a Voxel being a Member of a Specific Vascular Territory vs. the Other Territories.

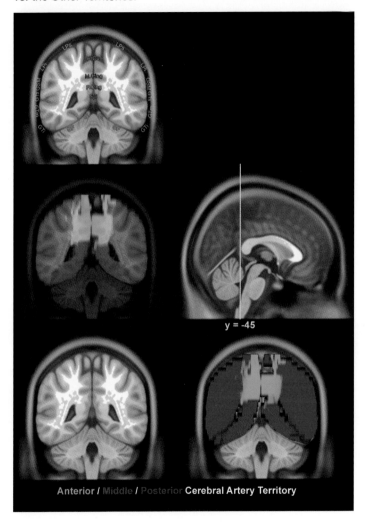

Anterior / Middle / Posterior Cerebral Artery Territory

Certainty Index (CI) Coronal (y = -50) MRI Maps: CI Reflects the Likelihood of a Voxel being a Member of a Specific Vascular Territory vs. the Other Territories.

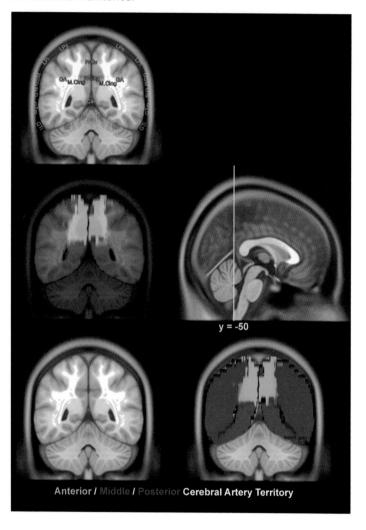

Anterior / Middle / Posterior Cerebral Artery Territory

Certainty Index (CI) Coronal (y = -55) MRI Maps: CI Reflects the Likelihood of a Voxel being a Member of a Specific Vascular Territory vs. the Other Territories.

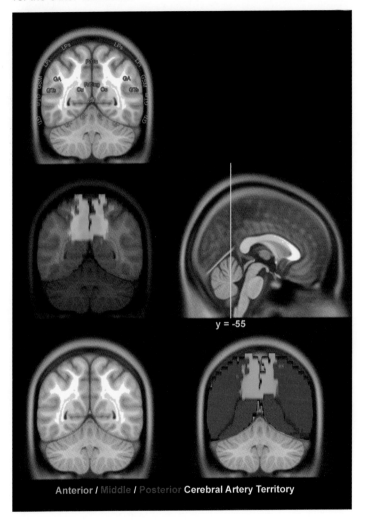

Anterior / Middle / Posterior Cerebral Artery Territory

Certainty Index (CI) Coronal (y = -60) MRI Maps: CI Reflects the Likelihood of a Voxel being a Member of a Specific Vascular Territory vs. the Other Territories.

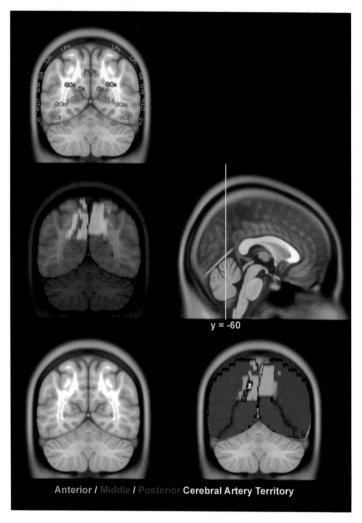

Anterior / Middle / Posterior **Cerebral Artery Territory**

Certainty Index (CI) Coronal (y = -65) MRI Maps: CI Reflects the Likelihood of a Voxel being a Member of a Specific Vascular Territory vs. the Other Territories.

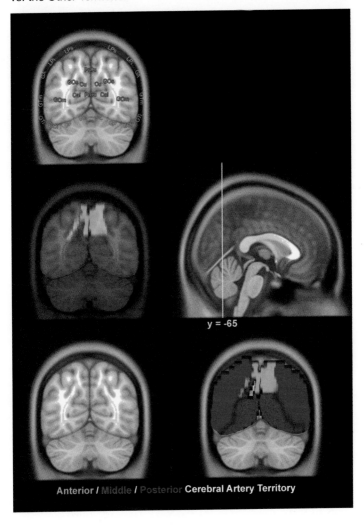

Certainty Index (CI) Coronal (y = -70) MRI Maps: CI Reflects the Likelihood of a Voxel being a Member of a Specific Vascular Territory vs. the Other Territories.

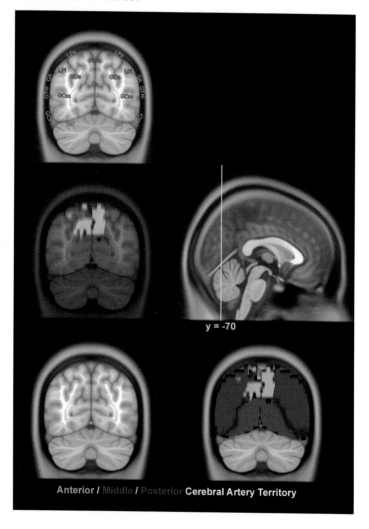

Anterior / Middle / Posterior **Cerebral Artery Territory**

Certainty Index (CI) Coronal (y = -75) MRI Maps: CI Reflects the Likelihood of a Voxel being a Member of a Specific Vascular Territory vs. the Other Territories.

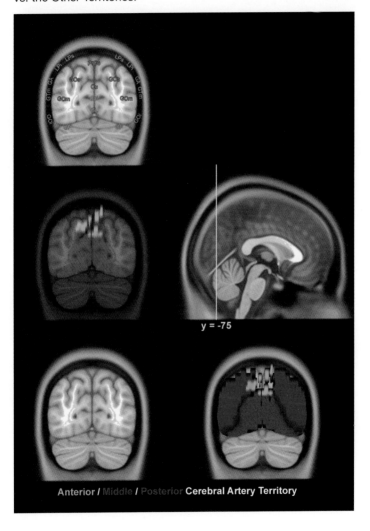

Anterior / Middle / Posterior **Cerebral Artery Territory**

Certainty Index (CI) Coronal (y = -80) MRI Maps: CI Reflects the Likelihood of a Voxel being a Member of a Specific Vascular Territory vs. the Other Territories.

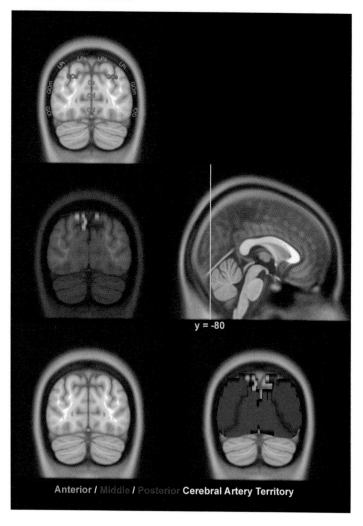

Anterior / Middle / Posterior **Cerebral Artery Territory**

PART

4

[Memo]

MR Angiography
and MR Venography

Eung Yeop Kim, MD, PhD

Figures

(1) (Contrast-enhanced) Intracranial and Extracranial Magnetic Resonance Angiography (MRA)

(2) Carotid / Vertebral Arterial Segments

(3) Time-of-Flight (TOF) Intracranial MRA

(4) Anterior Cerebral Artery and Middle Cerebral Artery: segments and branches

(5) Anterior Cerebral Artery and Middle Cerebral Artery: anteroposterior and lateral views

(6) Posterior Cerebral Artery: anteroposterior and lateral views

(7) Phase-contrast Venography: anteroposterior, lateral, oblique, and head-foot views

(1) (Contrast-enhanced) Intracranial and Extracranial MRA.

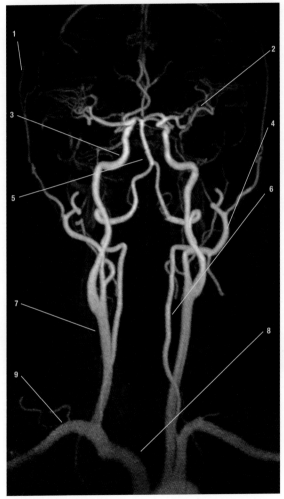

1. Superficial temporal artery
2. Middle cerebral artery
3. Internal carotid artery
4. External carotid artery
5. Basilar artery
6. Vertebral artery
7. Common carotid artery
8. Innominate artery
9. Subclavian artery

(2) Carotid / Vertebral Arterial Segments.

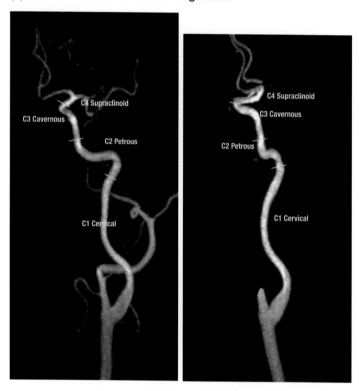

Cervical artery: Gibo Classification.

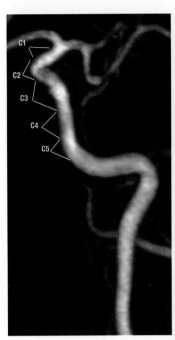

Cervical artery: Fischer
Classification.

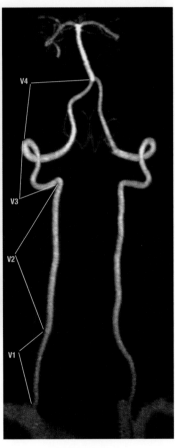

Vertebral artery.

(3) Time-of-Flight (TOF) Intracranial MRA.

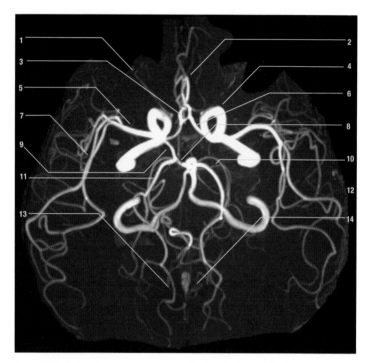

1. Ophthalmic artery
2. Anterior cerebral artery (A2 segment)
3. Anterior communicating artery
4. Internal carotid artery
5. Middle cerebral artery (M1 segment)
6. Anterior cerebral artery (A1 segment)
7. Middle cerebral artery (M2 segment)
8. Posterior cerebral artery (P1 segment)
9. Posterior communicating artery
10. Superior cerebellar artery
11. Posterior cerebral artery (P2 segment)
12. Temporal artery
13. Parieto-occipital artery
14. Calcarine artery

(4) Anterior Cerebral Artery and Middle Cerebral Artery:
segments and branches.

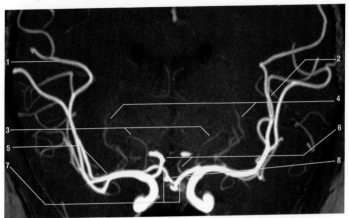

1. Middle cerebral artery
    (M3 segment)
2. Middle cerebral artery
    (M2 segment)
3. Anterior choroidal arteries
4. Lenticulostriate arteries
5. Middle cerebral artery
    (M1 segment)

6. Posterior communicating
    arteries
7. Anterior cerebral arteries
    (A1 segment)
8. Anterior communicating arteries

(5.1) Anterior Cerebral Artery and Middle Cerebral Artery: anteroposterior view.

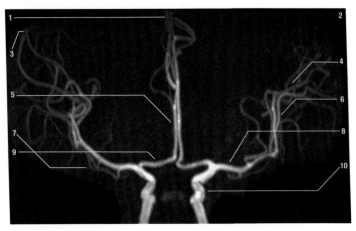

1. Callosmarginal artery
2. Pericallosal artery
3. Parietal artery
4. Middle cerebral artery (M3 segment)
5. Anterior cerebral artery (A2 segment)
6. Middle cerebral artery (M2 segment)
7. Anterior temporal artery
8. Middle cerebral artery (M1 segment)
9. Anterior cerebral artery (A1 segment)
10. Internal carotid artery

(5.2) Anterior Cerebral Artery and Middle Cerebral Artery: lateral view.

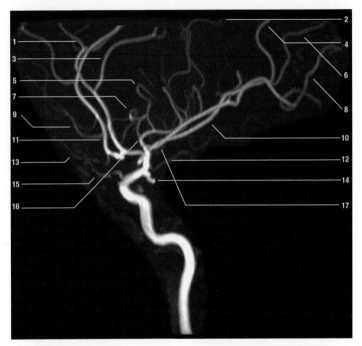

1. Callosmarginal artery
2. Central sulcus artery
3. Pericallosal artery
4. Anterior parietal artery
5. Precentral sulcus artery
6. Posterior parietal artery
7. Prefrontal artery
8. Angular artery
9. Polar frontal artery
10. Middle cerebral artery (M2 segment)

11. Anterior cerebral artery (A2 segment)
12. Anterior choroidal artery
13. Medial frontobasal artery
14. Posterior communicating artery
15. Ophthalmic artery
16. Superior division of middle cerebral artery
17. Inferior division of middle cerebral artery

(6.1) Posterior Cerebral Artery: anteroposterior view.

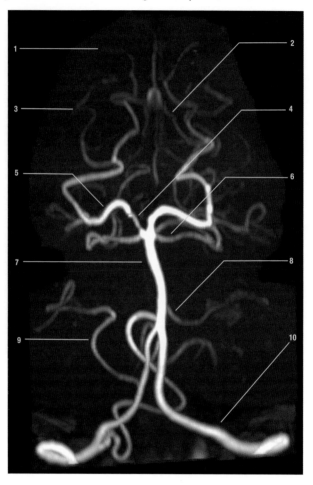

1. Parieto-occipital artery
2. Calcarine artery
3. Posterior temporal artery
4. P1 segment
5. P2 segment
6. Superior cerebellar artery
7. Basilar artery
8. Anterior inferior cerebellar artery
9. Posterior inferior cerebellar artery
10. Vertebral artery

(6.2) Posterior Cerebral Artery: lateral view.

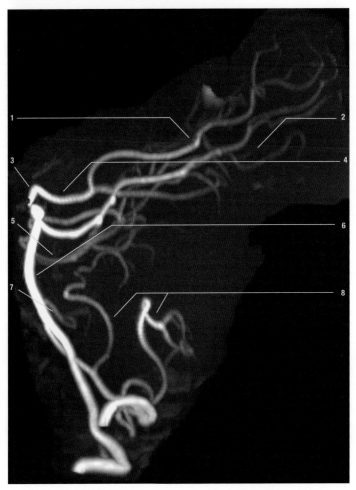

1. Parieto-occipital artery
2. Calcarine artery
3. P1 segment
4. P2 segment
5. Superior cerebellar artery
6. Basilar artery
7. Anterior inferior cerebellar artery
8. Posterior inferior cerebellar artery

(7.1) Phase-contrast Venography: anteroposterior view.

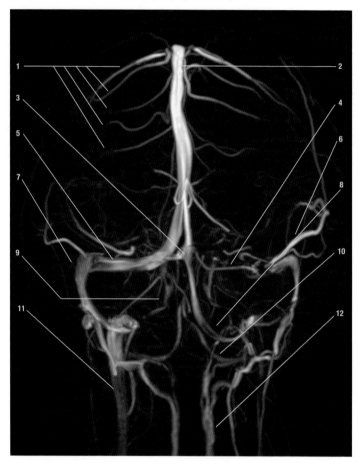

1. Superficial cortical veins
2. Superior sagittal sinus
3. Torcular Herophili
4. Transverse sinus (hypoplasia)
5. Transverse sinus
6. Vein of Labbe
7. Sigmoid sinus
8. Occipital sinus
9. Inferior petrosal sinus
10. Marginal sinus
11. Internal jugular vein
12. Vertebral venous plexus

(7.2) Phase-contrast Venography: lateral view.

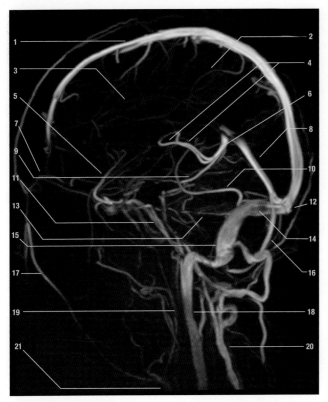

1. Superior sagittal sinus
2. Superficial cortical veins
3. Inferior sagittal sinus
4. Internal cerebral veins (Paired)
5. Superficial middle cerebral vein
6. Vein of Galen
7. Superior ophthalmic vein
8. Straight sinus
9. Basal vein of Rosenthal
10. Vein of Labbe
11. Inferior petrosal sinus
12. Torcular Herophili
13. Superior petrosal sinus
14. Transverse sinus
15. Sigmoid sinus
16. Occipital sinus
17. Facial vein
18. Internal jugular vein
19. Maxillary vein
20. Vertebral venous plexus
21. External jugular vein

(7.3) Phase-contrast Venography: oblique view.

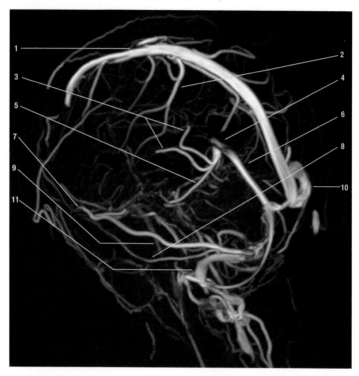

1. Superior sagittal sinus
2. Superficial cortical vein (vein of Trolard)
3. Internal cerebral veins (Paired)
4. Vein of Galen
5. Basal vein of Rosenthal
6. Straight sinus
7. Superficial middle cerebral vein
8. Vein of Labbe
9. Inferior petrosal sinus
10. Transverse sinus
11. Sigmoid sinus
12. Internal jugular vein

(7.4) Phase-contrast Venography: head-foot view I.

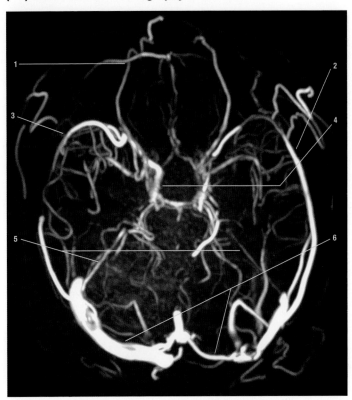

1. Superior ophthalmic vein
2. Superficial middle cerebral vein
3. Sphenoparietal sinus
4. Cavernous sinus
5. Superior petrosal sinus
6. Transverse sinus

(7.5) Phase-contrast Venography: head-foot view II.

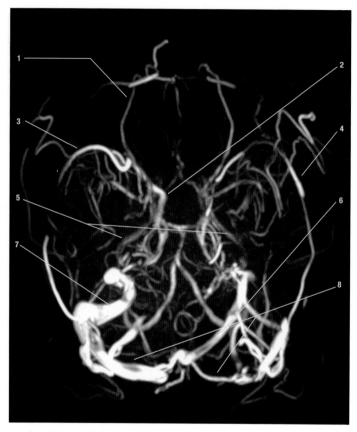

1. Superior ophthalmic vein
2. Cavernous sinus
3. Sphenoparietal sinus
4. Superficial middle cerebral vein
5. Inferior petrosal sinus
6. Occipital sinus
7. Sigmoid sinus
8. Transverse sinus

PART

5

[Memo]

Conventional Angiography

Woo-Keun Seo, MD, PhD

Figures

(1.1) Internal Carotid Artery (Lateral View).

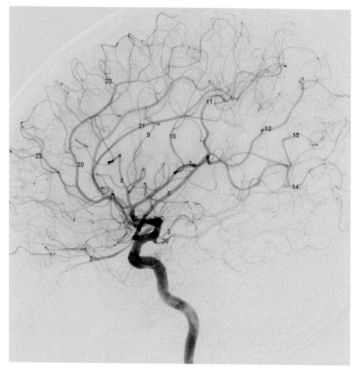

1. Internal carotid artery (C1–C5)
2. Ophthalmic artery
3. Anterior choroidal artery
4. Middle cerebral artery (M1)
5. Middle cerebral artery (superior branch)
8. Prefrontal artery
9. Precentral sulcal artery (pre-Rolandic artery)
10. Central sulcal artery (Rolandic artery)
11. Postcentral sulcal artery
12. Posterior parietal artery
13. Angular artery
14. Middle cerebral artery: posterior temporal branches
20. Callosomarginal artery
21. Pericallosal artery
22. Medial frontal artery(ies)
23. Paracentral artery

(1.2) Internal Carotid Artery (Anteroposterior View).

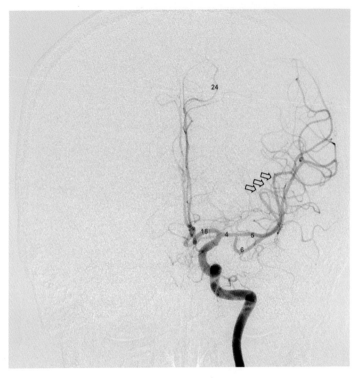

Arrows indicate M2 (insular) segment of the middle cerebral artery

4. Middle cerebral artery (M1)
5. Middle cerebral artery (superior branch)
6. Middle cerebral artery (inferior branch)

18. Anterior cerebral artery (A1)
24. Precuneal artery

(2.1) Extracranial-to-Intracranial Collateral Pathways Observed in the External Carotid Artery Angiogram in a Patient with Internal Carotid Artery Occlusion.

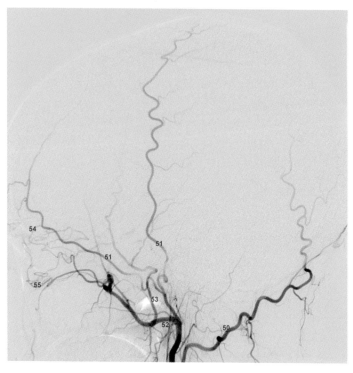

50. Occipital artery

51. Superficial temporal artery

52. Maxillary artery

53. Middle meningeal artery

54. Supraorbital artery

55. Infraorbital artery

(3.1) Anterior Cerebral Artery (Lateral View).

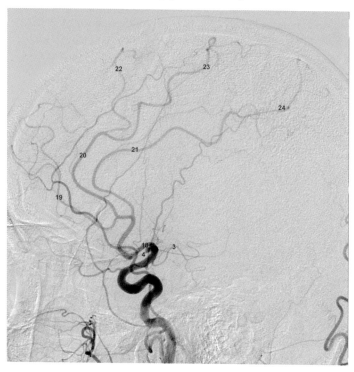

3. Anterior choroidal artery
4. Middle cerebral artery (M1)
18. Anterior cerebral artery (A1)
19. Frontal polar artery
(polar frontal artery)

20. Callosomarginal artery
21. Pericallosal artery
24. Precuneal artery

(3.2) Anterior Cerebral Artery (Anteroposterior View).

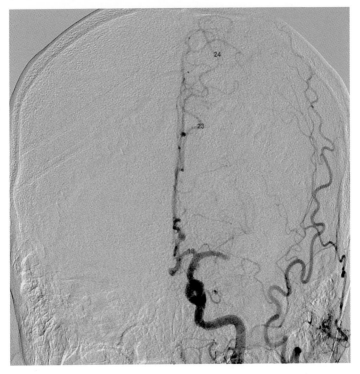

18. Anterior cerebral artery (A1)
23. Paracentral artery
24. Precuneal artery

(4.1) Middle Cerebral Artery (Lateral View).

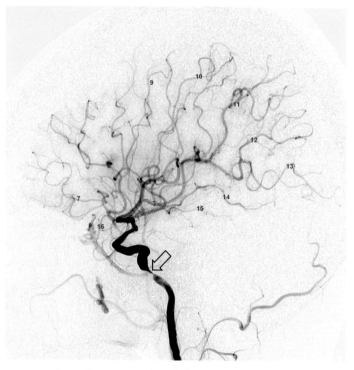

Arrow: focal severe stenosis in the petrous part of the
internal carotid artery

3. Anterior choroidal artery

7. Orbitofrontal artery

8. Prefrontal artery

9. Precentral sulcal artery
(Pre-Rolandic artery)

10. Central sulcal artery
(Rolandic artery)

11. Postcentral sulcal artery

12. Posterior parietal artery

13. Angular artery

14. Middle cerebral artery:
posterior temporal branches

15. Middle cerebral artery:
middle temporal branches

16. Middle cerebral artery:
anterior temporal branches

(4.2) Middle Cerebral Artery (Anteroposterior View).

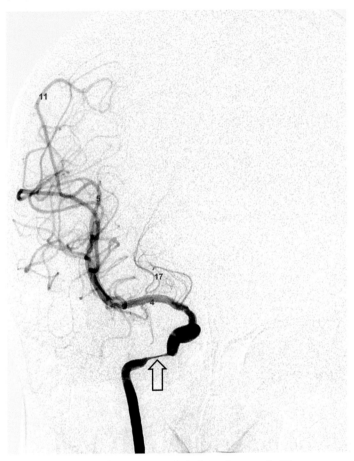

Arrow: focal severe stenosis in the petrous part of the
internal carotid artery

4. Middle cerebral artery (M1)

5. Middle cerebral artery
   (superior branch)

11. Postcentral sulcal artery

17. Lenticulostriate artery

(5.1) Distal Vertebral / Basilar / Posterior Cerebral Artery (Lateral View).

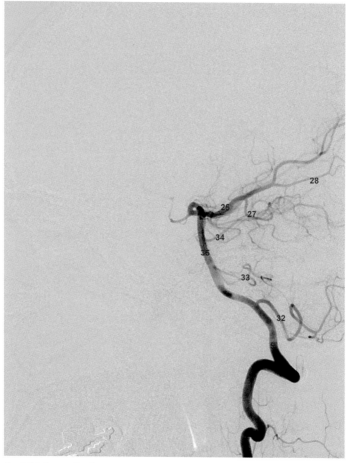

5. Middle cerebral artery (superior branch)

25. Posterior cerebral artery

27. Posterior cerebral artery: anterior temporal artery

28. Posterior cerebral artery: posterior temporal artery

32. Posterior inferior cerebellar artery

33. Anterior inferior cerebellar artery

34. Superior cerebellar artery

35. Basilar artery

(5.2) Distal Vertebral / Basilar / Posterior Cerebral Artery (Anteroposterior View).

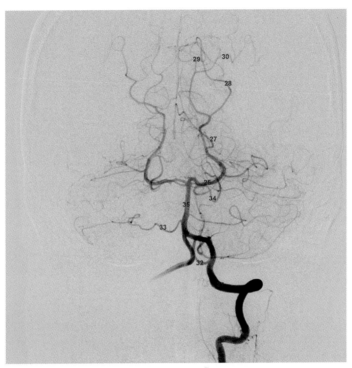

25. Posterior cerebral artery

27. Posterior cerebral artery: anterior temporal artery

28. Posterior cerebral artery: posterior temporal artery

29. Calarine artery

30. Parietooccipital artery

31. Vertebral artery

32. Posterior inferior cerebellar artery

33. Anterior inferior cerebellar artery

34. Superior cerebellar artery

35. Basilar artery

(6.1) Early Venous Phase Internal Carotid Artery Angiogram (Lateral View).

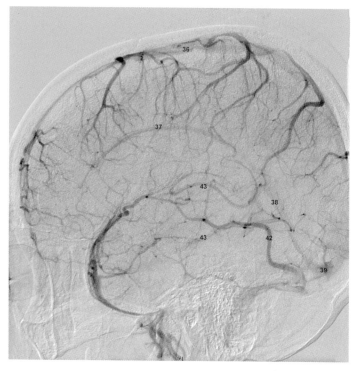

36. Superior sagittal sinus
37. Inferior sagittal sinus
38. Straight sinus

39. Torcular Herophili
42. Vein of Labbe
43. Internal cerebral vein

(6.2) Late Venous Phase Internal Carotid Artery Angiogram (Lateral View).

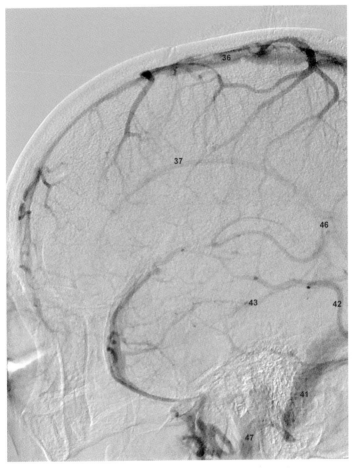

36. Superior sagittal sinus
37. Inferior sagittal sinus
41. Sigmoid sinus
42. Vein of Labbe

43. Internal cerebral vein
46. Vein of Galen
47. Internal jugular vein
48. Vein of Trolard

(6.3) Venous Phase Internal Carotid Artery Angiogram (AnteroPosterior View).

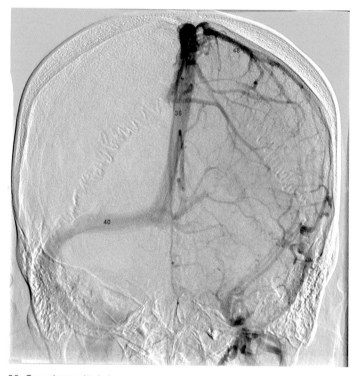

36. Superior sagittal sinus
40. Transverse sinus
48. Vein of Trolard

(7) Modified Thrombolysis in Cerebral Infarction (mTICI) Score, which ranges from 0 (no reperfusion) to 3 (complete reperfusion), after endovascular thrombectomy for proximal middle cerebral artery (MCA) occlusion.

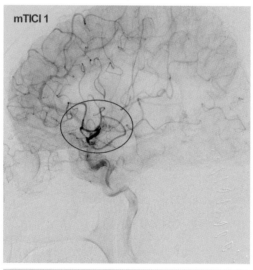

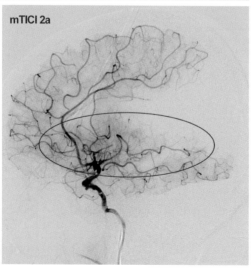

mTICI 1: Localized arterial contrast filling (red ellipse) in the late arterial / capillary phase

mTICI 2a: >50% perfusion defect remaining in the MCA superior division area. Red ellipses indicate the areas supplied by the inferior division of the MCA.

mTICI 2b: Delayed and reduced cerebral perfusion in the distal portion of the MCA (arrows).

mTICI 3: Full recanalization

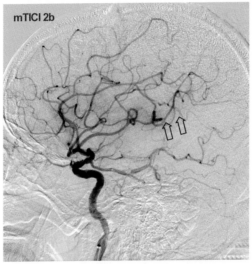

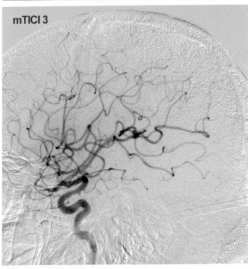

(8) Cervical Carotid Artery Diseases.

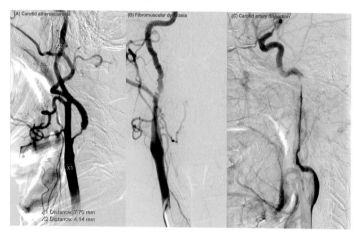

(A) Carotid atherosclerosis   (B) Fibromuscular dysplasia   (C) Carotid artery dissection

(A) Segmental stenosis due to atherosclerotic plaque

(B) "Stroke-of-beads" sign in fibromuscular dysplasia

(C) "String sign" in arterial dissection

PART
6

[Memo]

High-resolution Vessel Wall MRI

Jong-Won Chung, MD, PhD;
Oh Young Bang, MD, PhD

Black-blood High-resolution Vessel Wall MRI Protocol

(1) Axial and sagittal proton-density: TR/TE = 2150/12.5 msec, echo train length (ETL) = 10, slice thickness = 2 mm, flip angle = 90°, matrix = 280 × 280, FOV = 14 cm, no. of average (NEX) = 2

(2) Axial and sagittal T2-weighted images: TR/TE = 2150/100 msec, ETL = 10, slice thickness = 2 mm, flip angle = 90°, matrix = 280 × 280, FOV = 14 cm, NEX = 2

(3) Sagittal T1 fluid-attenuated inversion recovery, pre- and post-contrast: TR/TE = 2100/10 msec, ETL = 6, slice thickness = 2 mm, flip angle = 90°, matrix = 280 × 280, FOV = 14 cm, NEX = 2

(4) Axial post-contrast 3D T1-weighted volumetric isotropic turbo spin echo (TSE) acquisition (VISTA): TR/TE = 350/20 msec, TSE factor = 25, 0.5 mm isotropic voxel, flip angle = 90°, matrix = 360 × 360, FOV = 18 cm, NEX = 2.

Table 1. Summary of High-resolution Vessel Wall MRI Findings

	Atherosclerosis	**Moyamoya Disease**
Location	Any artery	Terminal ICA, proximal MCA, ACA
Cross sectional shape	Eccentric plaque	Concentric narrowing
Enhancement	Eccentric enhance at symptomatic site	Concentric enhance at the site of progressive stenosis
T1 hyperintensity	Lipid (isointense), fibrous tissue (isointense), calcification (hypointense)	Isointense
T2 intensity	Lipid (hypointense), fibrous tissue (isointense), calcification (hypointense)	Isointense
Remodeling pattern	Usually positive remodeling, but less prominent in branch atheromatous disease	Negative remodeling
Others	Intraplaque hemorrhage	Basal collaterals
Progress	Regression with statin (70%), progression without medication	Stationary or progression

Abbreviations: RCVS, reversible cerebral vasoconstriction syndrome; ICA, internal carotid artery; MCA, middle cerebral artery; ACA, anterior cerebral artery; VA, vertebral artery; BA, basilar artery.

Dissection	Vasculitis	RCVS
Any artery (frequent in VA, ACA, BA)	Medium- to small-sized vessels	Medium- to small-sized vessels (distal -to proximal)
Eccentric or combined	Concentric stenosis	Concentric stenosis
Diffuse enhancement due to inflammation during weeks after dissection	Concentric enhancement during active stage	None
Intramural hematoma (hyperintense)	Isointense	Isointense
Variable	Isointense	Isointense
Dependent on stage (positive remodeling with mural hematoma, but normal or negative remodeling during chronic stage)	Variable	Negative remodeling
Intimal flap, double lumen, intramural hematoma, or aneurysmal dilatation	Exclusive diagnosis	Exclusive diagnosis
Resolution (37%-75%)	Resolution with medication	Spontaneous/with medication reversibility

Abbreviations

ACA: anterior cerebral artery

BA: basilar artery

CT: computed tomography

DWI: diffusion-weighted imaging

HR-MRI: high-resolution magnetic resonance imaging

ICA: internal carotid artery

ICAS-BOD: intracranial atherosclerotic stroke - branch occlusive disease

ICAS-NBOD: intracranial atherosclerotic stroke - non-branch occlusive disease

MCA: middle cerebral artery

MTT: mean transit time

PCA: posterior cerebral artery

PD: proton-density

PWI: perfusion-weighted imaging

TOF-MRA: time-of-flight magnetic resonance angiography

TFCA: transfemoral cerebral angiography

Figures

(1) ICAS-BOD Type Acute MCA Infarction

(2) ICAS-BOD Type Acute BA Infarction

(3) ICAS-NBOD Type Acute MCA Infarction; Before: Statin Treatment

(4) ICAS-NBOD Type Acute MCA Infarction: 6 months after 20 mg Rosuvastatin Treatment

(5) Imaging Assessment of Intracranial Stent Patency

(6) Moyamoya Disease

(7) Intracranial Artery Dissection

(8) Primary Angiitis of the Central Nervous System (Pre- and Post-steroid Treatment)

(9) Reversible Cerebral Vasoconstriction Syndrome (Pre- and Post-nimodipine Treatment)

(1) ICAS-BOD Type Acute MCA Infarction: M/76 with sudden onset right side weakness.

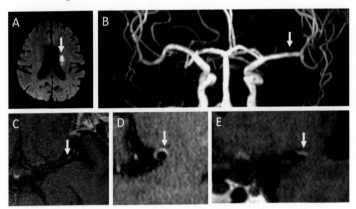

A. DWI: acute infarction in the left corona radiata.

B. TOF-MRA: subtle focal narrowing of the left distal MCA.

C. HR-MRI T1 enhance (axial): diffuse enhancement of the left MCA.

D. HR-MRI T1 enhance (sagittal): enhancing plaque predominantly in the upper portion.

E. HR-MRI T1 enhance (coronal): enhancing plaque predominantly in the upper portion.

(2) ICAS-BOD type acute BA infarction: M/78 with dysarthria and right side weakness.

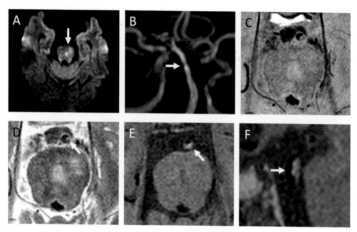

A. DWI: acute infarction in the left pons.

B. TOF-MRA: focal stenosis in the distal BA.

C. HR-MRI PD-VISTA (axial): eccentric plaque in the postero-lateral part of the BA.

D. HR-MRI T2 (axial): eccentric plaque in the postero-lateral part of the BA.

E. HR-MRI T1 enhance (axial): enhancement of the atherosclerotic plaque.

F. HR-MRI T1 enhance (sagittal): longitudinal enhancement of the atherosclerotic plaque in the posterior wall of the BA.

(3) ICAS-NBOD Type Acute MCA infarction; Before Statin Treatment: F/65 with sudden onset right side weakness.

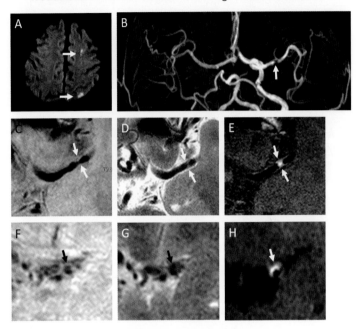

A. DWI: acute infarction in the left cortical boarder zone.

B. TOF: focal severe stenosis in the distal MCA.

C. HR-MRI PD vista (axial): eccentric plaque in the MCA.

D. HR-MRI T2 (axial): eccentric plaque in the MCA.

E. HR-MRI T1 enhance (axial): enhancement of the atherosclerotic plaque.

F. HR-MRI PD-VISTA (sagittal): eccentric plaque in the upper portion of the MCA.

G. HR-MRI T2 (sagittal): eccentric plaque in the upper portion of the MCA.

H. HR-MRI T1 enhance (axial): enhancement of the atherosclerotic plaque.

(4) ICAS-NBOD Type Acute MCA Infarction, 6 months after 20 mg Rosuvastatin Treatment; please compare with the corresponding figures in the left page.

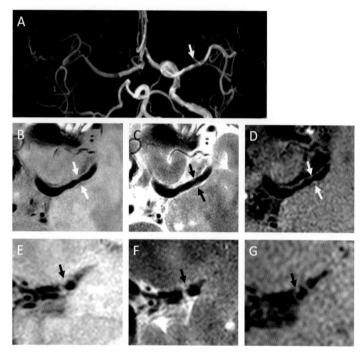

A. TOF: focal mild stenosis in the distal MCA: improved.

B. HR-MRI PD-VISTA (axial): eccentric plaque in the MCA.

C. HR-MRI T2 (axial): eccentric plaque in the MCA.

D. HR-MRI T1 enhance (axial): diffuse enhancement of the atherosclerotic plaque: improved.

E. HR-MRI PD-VISTA (sagittal): small eccentric plaque in the upper portion of the MCA.

F. HR-MRI T2 (sagittal): eccentric plaque in the upper portion of the MCA.

G. HR-MRI T1 enhance (axial): focal enhancement of the atherosclerotic plaque.

(5) Imaging Assessment of intracranial Stent Patency: M/75 with recurrent transient monocular blindness.

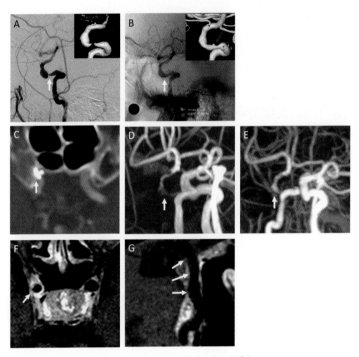

A. TFCA: severe focal stenosis in the right distal ICA.

B. TFCA: improved right distal ICA stenosis after stenting.

C. Non-contrast CT: artifact due to the stent.

D. TOF-MRA: artifact due to the stent.

E. Contrast enhanced MRA: artifact due to the stent

F. HR-MRI T1 (axial): no evidence of instent restenosis.

G. HR-MRI T1 (3D-reconstructed image).

(6) Moyamoya Disease: F/30 with recurrent right side weakness.

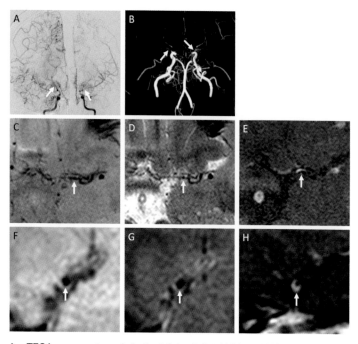

A. TFCA: severe stenosis in the bilateral distal ICA and MCA with basal collaterals.

B. TOF-MRA: occlusion of the right distal ICA and severe stenosis in the left distal ICA / MCA

C. HR-MRI PD-VISTA (axial): shrinked MCA with negative remodeling and basal collaterals.

D. HR-MRI T2 (axial): shrinked MCA with negative remodeling and basal collaterals.

E. HR-MRI T1 enhance (axial): focal enhancement in the left MCA.

F. HR-MRI PD-VISTA (sagittal): shrinked MCA with negative remodeling

G. HR-MRI T2 (sagittal): shrinked MCA with negative remodeling.

H. HR-MRI T1 enhance (axial): focal enhancement in the left MCA.

(7) Intracranial Artery Dissection: F/67 with sudden onset global aphasia after falling down.

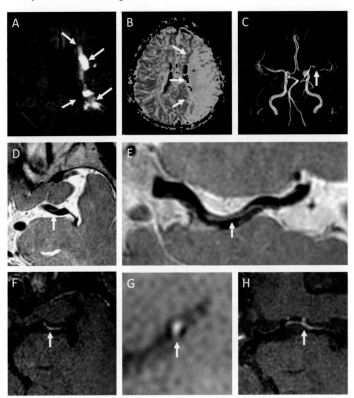

A. DWI: acute infarction in the internal boarder zone.

B. PWI (MTT): perfusion delay in the left MCA territory.

C. TOF-MRA: tandem occlusion in the left MCA.

D. HR-MRI PD-VISTA (axial): intimal flap in the MCA.

E. HR-MRI PD-VISTA (Teracon 3D recon): intimal flap along the MCA.

F. HR-MRI T1 enhance (axial): diffuse enhancement of the intimal flap.

G. HR-MRI T1 enhance (sagittal): enhancing intimal flap in the MCA.

(8) Primary Angiitis of the Central Nervous System (Pre- and Post-steroid Treatment): F/38 with severe headache and transient aphasia.

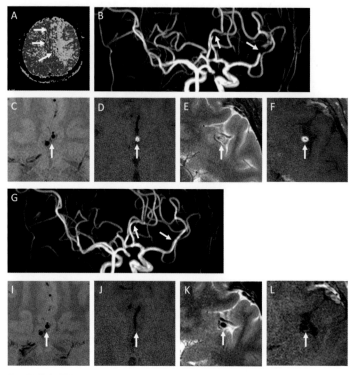

A. PWI (MTT): perfusion delay in the left ACA and MCA territory.

B. TOF-MRA: tandem occlusion in the left ACA and MCA M2 branch

C. HR-MRI PD-VISTA (axial): thickening of the ACA.

D. HR-MRI T1 enhance (axial): concentric enhancement of the left ACA.

E. HR-MRI PD-VISTA (axial): thickening of the MCA.

F. HR-MRI T1 enhance (axial): concentric enhancement of the left MCA.

G-L. When compared with the corresponding figures (B-F, respectively), definite improvement in the wall thickening and enhancement is observed after steroid treatment for 3 months.

(9) Reversible Cerebral Vasoconstriction Syndrome (Pre- and Post-nimodipine Treatment): F/29 with headache after uterine myomectomy.

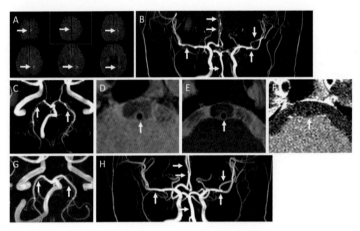

A. DWI: multiple acute ischemic lesions in the left ACA and MCA territories.

B. TOF-MRA: multiple intracranial arterial stenosis.

C. TOF-MRA: focal stenosis in the bilateral PCAs.

D. HR-MRI PD-VISTA (axial): concentric narrowing of the BA.

E. HR-MRI T2 (axial): concentric narrowing of the BA.

F. HR-MRI T1 enhance (axial): concentric narrowing of the BA without enhancement.

G. TOF-MRA: complete regression of the bilateral PCA stenosis after nimodipine treatment for 2 months.

H. TOF-MRA: complete regression of multiple intracranial arterial stenosis after nimodipine treatment for 2 months.

PART

7

[Memo]

Visual Estimation of Leukoaraisosis Burden

Wi-Sun Ryu, MD, PhD; Dong-Eog Kim, MD, PhD

(A) A Visual Garding System for White Matter Hyperintensity (WMH)

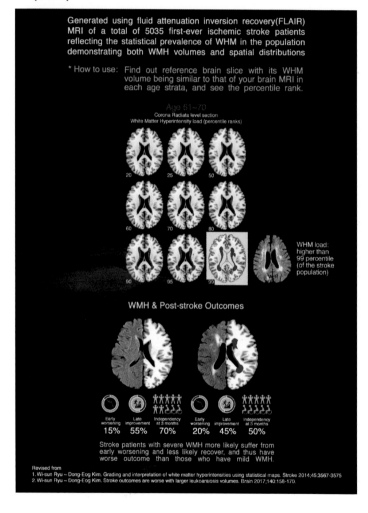

Generated using fluid attenuation inversion recovery(FLAIR) MRI of a total of 5035 first-ever ischemic stroke patients reflecting the statistical prevalence of WHM in the population demonstrating both WMH volumes and spatial distributions

* How to use: Find out reference brain slice with its WHM volume being similar to that of your brain MRI in each age strata, and see the percentile rank.

Age 51~70
Corona Radiata level section
White Matter Hyperintensity load (percentile ranks)

20   25   50

60   70   80

90   95   99

WHM load: higher than 99 percentile (of the stroke population)

WMH & Post-stroke Outcomes

Early worsening	Late improvement	Independency at 3 months	Early worsening	Late improvement	Independency at 3 months
15%	55%	70%	20%	45%	50%

Stroke patients with severe WMH more likely suffer from early worsening and less likely recover, and thus have worse outcome than those who have mild WMH.

Revised from
1. Wi-sun Ryu ~ Dong-Eog Kim. Grading and interpretation of white matter hyperintensities using statistical maps. Stroke 2014;45:3567-3575
2. Wi-sun Ryu ~ Dong-Eog Kim. Stroke outcomes are worse with larger leukoaraiosis volumes. Brain 2017;140:158-170.

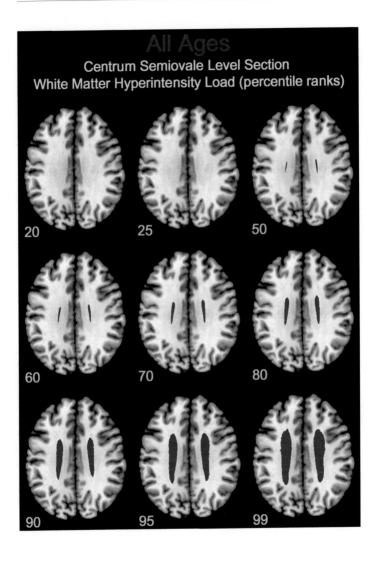

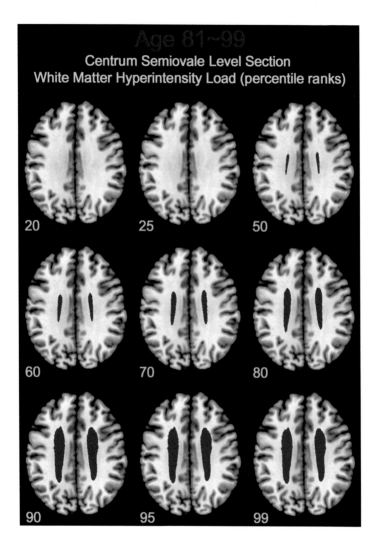

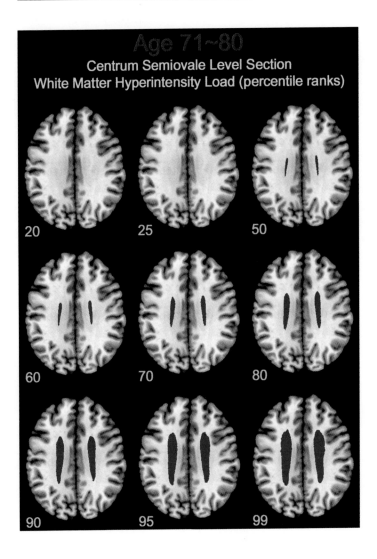

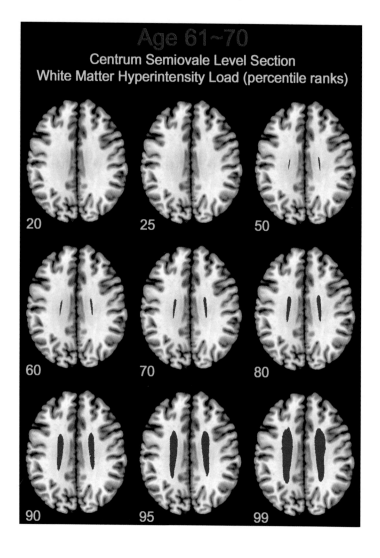

Age 61~70
Centrum Semiovale Level Section
White Matter Hyperintensity Load (percentile ranks)

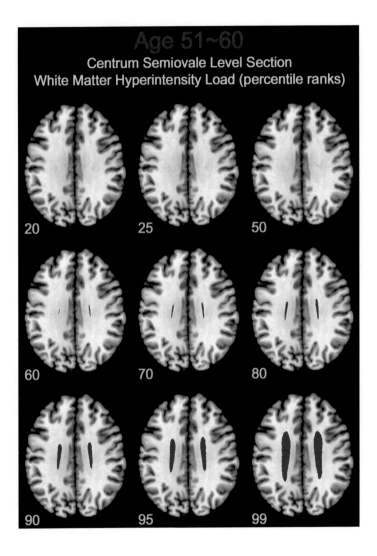

Age 51~60
Centrum Semiovale Level Section
White Matter Hyperintensity Load (percentile ranks)

20 25 50

60 70 80

90 95 99

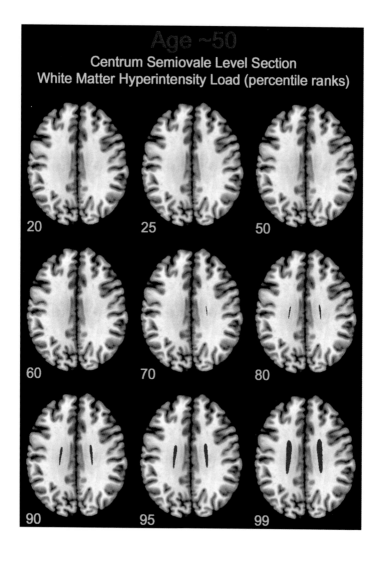

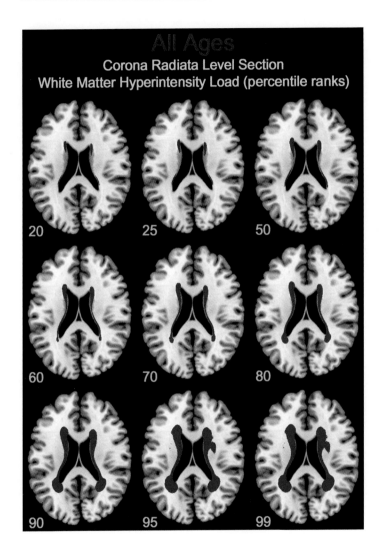

All Ages
Corona Radiata Level Section
White Matter Hyperintensity Load (percentile ranks)

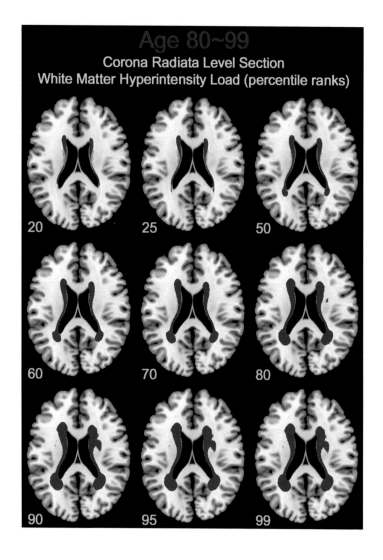

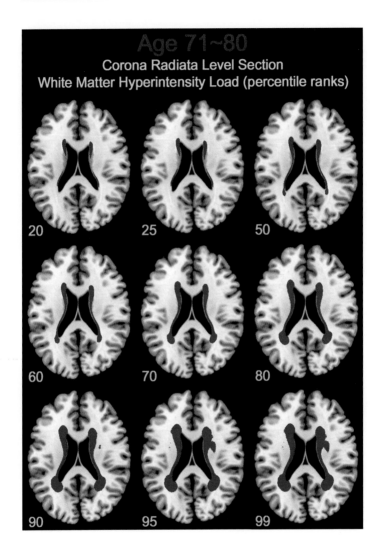

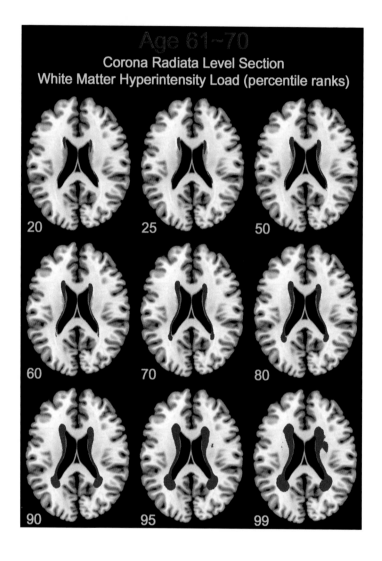

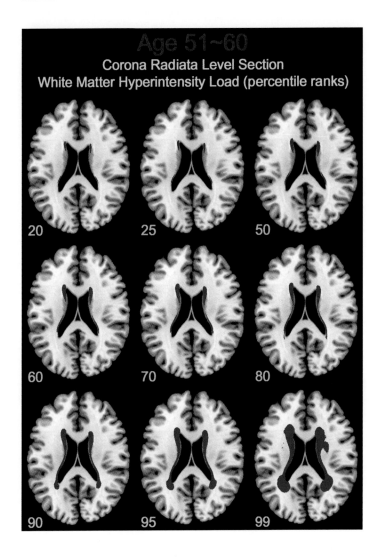

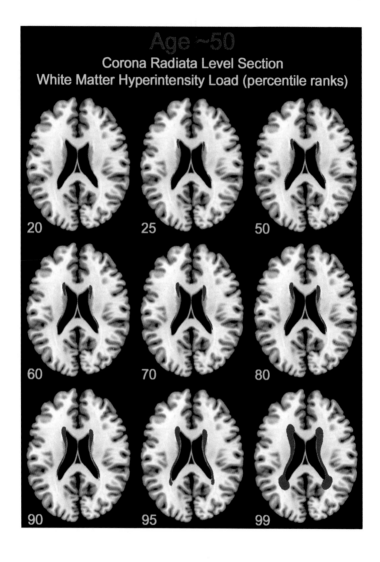

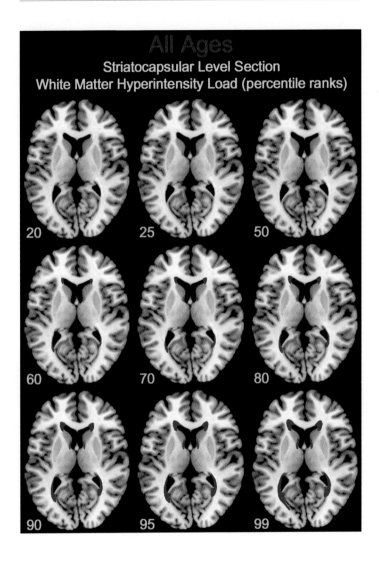

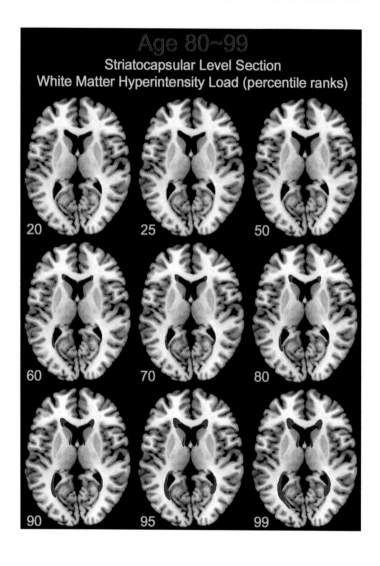

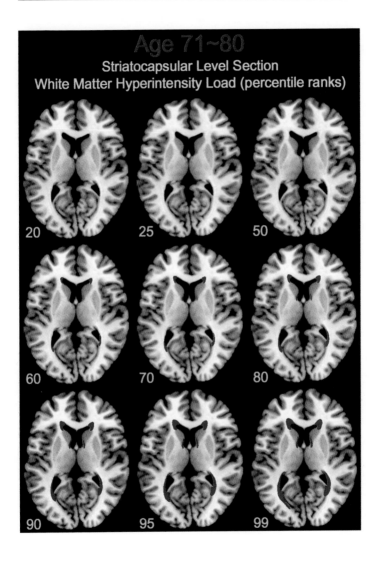

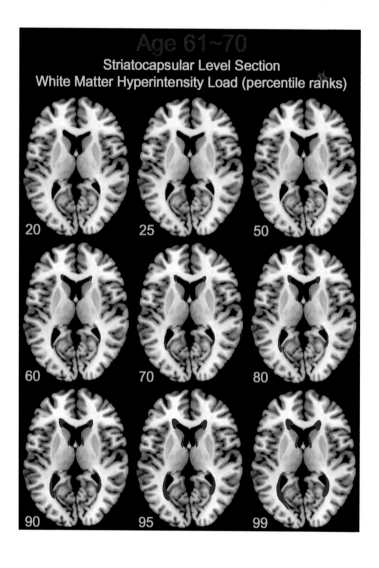

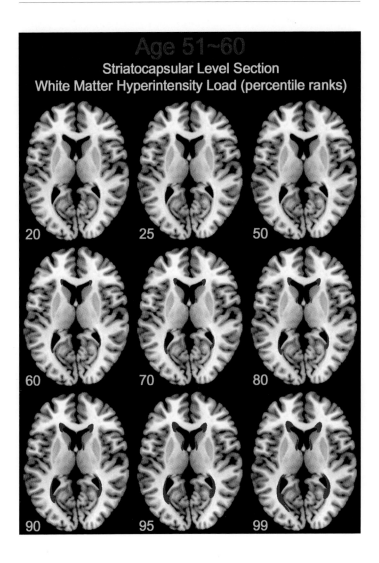

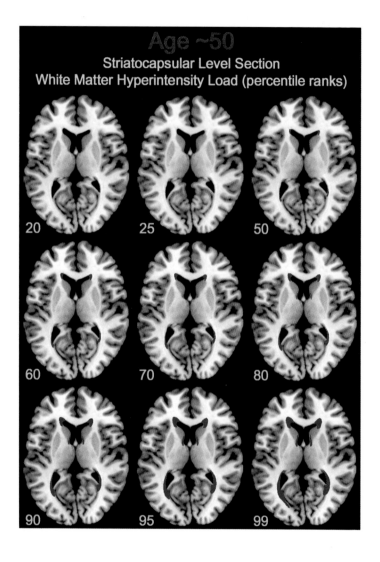

PART
8

[Memo]

Appendix

I.   Proportion of patients achieving modified Rankin Scale score of 0 – 2 at discharge, stratified by age and initial NIHSS score after intravenous thrombolysis.

II. Symptomatic intracerebral hemorrhage risk, stratified by age and initial NIHSS score after intravenous thrombolysis.

III. Visual estimation of infarct volume for decision making in thrombectomy cases.

I. Proportion of Patients Achieving Modified Rankin Scale Score of 0 – 2 at Discharge, stratified by Age and Initial NIHSS Score after Intravenous Thrombolysis.

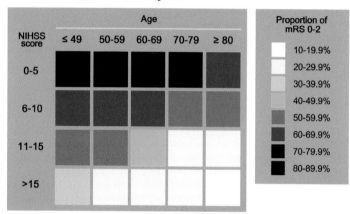

II. Symptomatic Intracerebral Hemorrhage Risk, stratified by Age and Initial NIHSS Score after Intravenous Thrombolysis

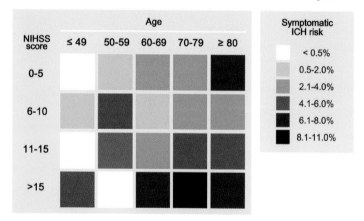

Pictures (courtesy of Pf. Keun-Sik Hong, Ilsan Paik Hospital, Inje University, Korea & Pf. Sung-Il Sohn, Keimyung University Dongsan Medical Center, Korea), derived from Hye Jung Lee *et al.* Simple estimates of symptomatic intracranial hemorrhage risk and outcome after intravenous thrombolysis using age and stroke severity. *Stroke* 2017;19:229-231.

III. Visual Estimation of Infarct Volume for Decision Making in Thrombectomy Cases.

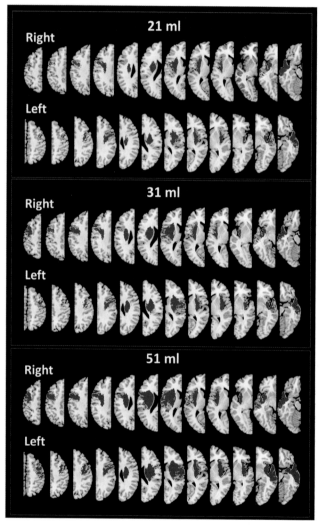

from Dong-Eog Kim *et al.* Estimation of acute infarct volume with reference maps: a simple visual tool for decision making in thrombectomy cases. *Journal of Stroke;* 2019; 21:69-77.

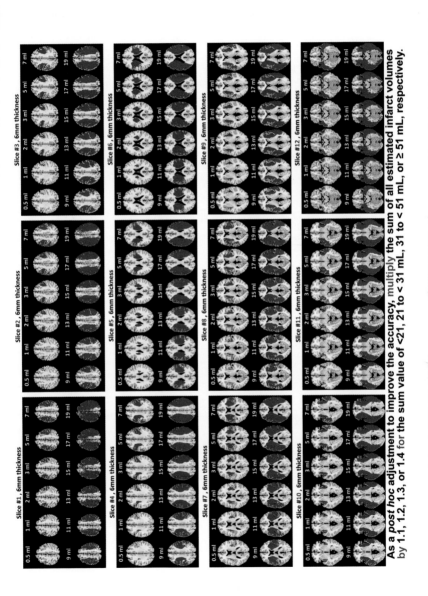

As a *post hoc* adjustment to improve the accuracy, multiply the sum of all estimated infarct volumes by 1.1, 1.2, 1.3, or 1.4 for the sum value of <21, 21 to < 31 mL, 31 to < 51 mL, or ≥ 51 mL, respectively.

[Memo]

Index